VOGUE

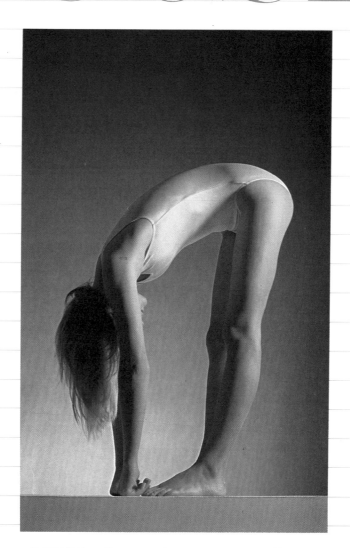

EXERCISE
BOOK

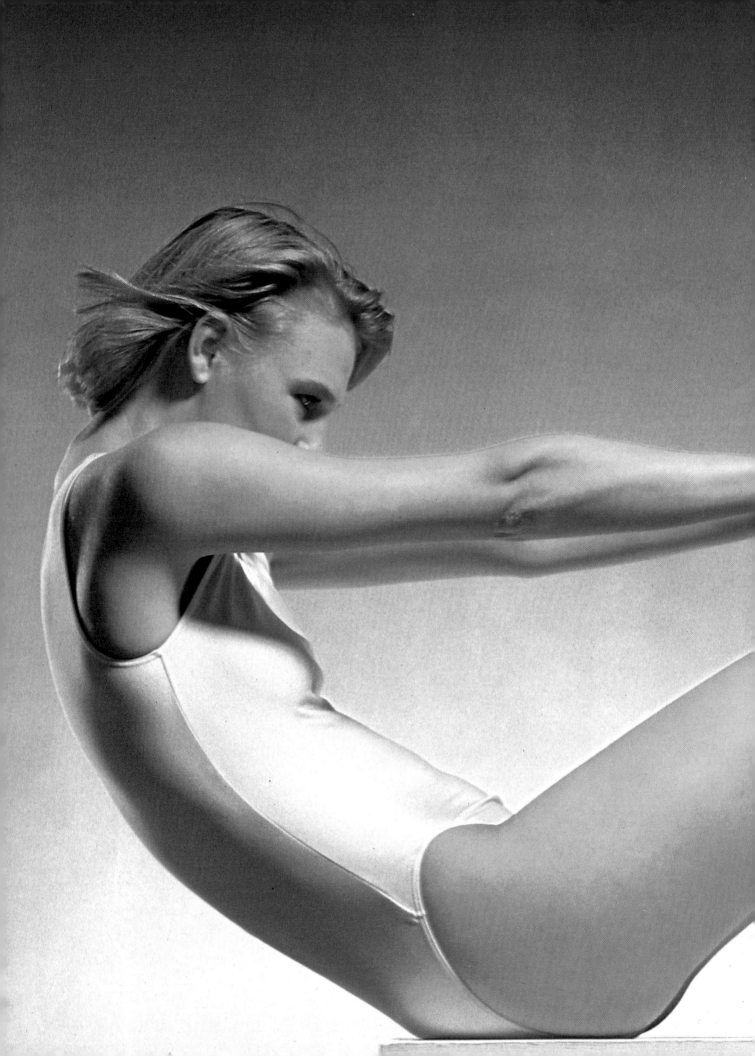

VOGUE
EXERCISE BOOK

General Editor
Deborah Hutton

Octopus Books

The contributors

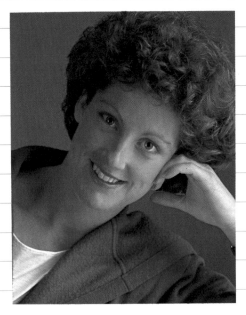 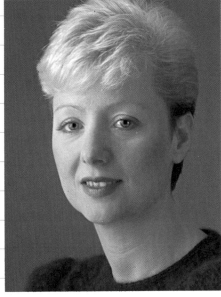 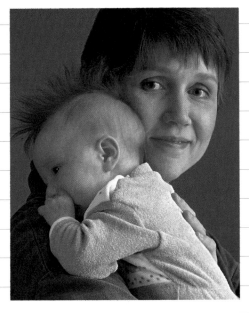

DEBORAH HUTTON devised the concept for the book, wrote and edited it. She has an honours degree in English from York University and gained a job on *Vogue* after entering their annual talent competition in 1979. She has been writing health features for the magazine for 5 years and is the author of *Vogue Complete Beauty*.

EILEEN FAIRBANE devised the major part of the 24-week programme, the jazz, pre-ski and therapeutic sections. A jazz dancer, who trained with Matt Mattox and Molly Molloy, she is also interested in classical Greek ballet, folk dance and oriental movement. She is a qualified beauty therapist and trained aromatherapist and has studied shiatsu (acupressure), macrobiotics and Feldenkrais work. Believing strongly that exercise and movement should be seen in the context of the whole person, she has developed her own back-to-basics course, which aims at gently introducing the body to more vigorous forms of exercise. She teaches stretch and aerobics at The Dance Centre, Covent Garden and The Pineapple Studio, South Kensington, and has produced her own exercise tape cassette and record. She also contributed to the Autumn/Winter 1982 issue of *Health & Beauty in Vogue*.

BARBARA DALE devised the pre- and post-natal exercise programme. She trained from the age of 11 in all aspects of Dance at the Arts Educational Trust in Hertfordshire, and later studied the Martha Graham technique at the London School of Contemporary Dance. She then followed a teacher training course specializing in movement at Goldsmith's College, London University. A further course in the Mensedieck Method of Body Education enabled her to combine all these influences into the Bodywork method of exercise, which she now teaches at her own Bodyworkshop Exercise Studio in London. Her main concern is to promote exercise as a natural prerequisite to good health for all ages and to ensure the highest standards in exercise teaching. Classes include Bodywork, Relaxation, Yoga, Ante- and Post-Natal Exercises and teacher training courses. Barbara is co-author of *Simple Movement* (John Murray, 1980) and *Exercises for Childbirth* (Century, 1982), and a contributor to *The Health and Fitness Handbook* (Sphere, 1981). She devised the exercise section for *Vogue Complete Beauty* (Octopus, 1982) and has often contributed special exercise features to *Vogue* magazine.

This book first published 1984 by
Octopus Books Limited
59 Grosvenor Street
London W1.

ISBN 0 7064 2077 2

Printed by Gráficas Estella SA,
Spain

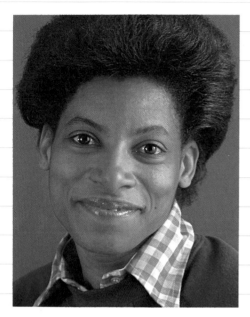

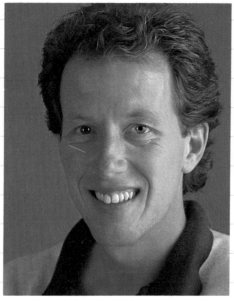

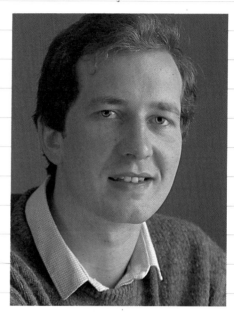

CYLE POLLARD devised the Rock and Roll section and the special preparatory exercises which appear in week 19 of the general programme. She was born in Chicago and has taught and performed in the Middle East, West Germany, Holland and Paris. She has a particular interest in American jazz dance and has established numerous projects in the London area. She is the new Director of the Footwork Dance Studio in London.

CHRISTOPHER CONNOLLY produced most of the Feldenkrais-based awareness movements for the programme, plus many of the therapeutic exercises, and helped to check the text. He has a bachelors degree from the University of Michigan and a masters degree from Antioch University, Ohio and produced his thesis on the use of visual imagery to improve the function of the body. He trained with Dr Moshe Feldenkrais in Israel and the USA and is the only qualified teacher of his method in the UK. He is also trained in psychosynthesis and teaches at the Psychosynthesis and Education Trust. In 1979, he co-founded the Sporting Bodymind, an organization teaching professional and amateur sportspeople techniques for improving their body/mind coordination. He is co-author of *Sporting Body, Sporting Mind,* an athlete's guide to mental training, published by Cambridge University Press in Spring 1984, and has helped compile several movement sequences for *Vogue.*

TONY LYCHOLAT acted as general consultant throughout the compiling of the book and helped to check the text. He has an honours degree in Human Movement, specializing in sports science, from the University of Kent and is currently completing a MSc degree at King's College in London, where he is studying Human and Applied Physiology. A keen runner himself, he is an athletics coach who regularly lectures on exercise and training theory, a founder member of the Central Affiliation of Professional Exercise Teachers and Fitness Advisor to Barbara Dale's Bodyworkshop in Bayswater, London. Recently, he has become involved in trying to raise standards of exercise teaching and in increasing the degree of communication between different exercise teachers and dance studios.

Much help was received during the compiling of this book, but we are, in particular, grateful to Beatrix Miller, Vogue Editor-in-Chief, and Alex Kroll, Vogue Books Editor, for their enthusiasm and support; Penny Summers and Marie-Louise Avery of Octopus Books for their care with the manuscript and its presentation; John Hind, Vogue Art Editor, for his work on the design; Paul Manley, for checking some of the exercises, Christopher Nixon, for advising on the pre-ski section, Myriam Pfeffer, for contributing some of the Feldenkrais work and Joanna Gibbon, Vogue Editorial Assistant, for her help with every detail.

CONTENTS

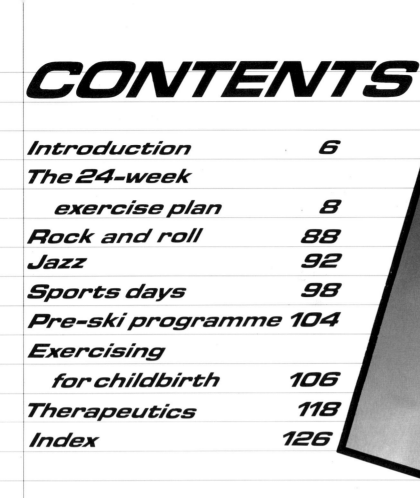

INTRODUCTION

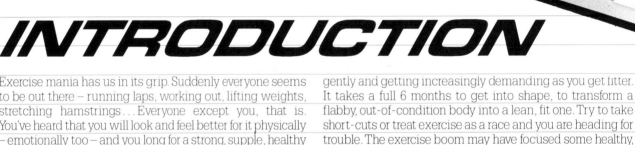

Exercise mania has us in its grip. Suddenly everyone seems to be out there – running laps, working out, lifting weights, stretching hamstrings…Everyone except you, that is. You've heard that you will look and feel better for it physically – emotionally too – and you long for a strong, supple, healthy body. But it seems impossible to get started.

The sheer difficulty of knowing how and where to start can seem daunting enough. As awareness of fitness has increased, so ways of getting fit have multiplied. There are hundreds of different methods, each claiming to be better than the next. Who is right? What is best? Running or swimming? Swimming or yoga? Straightforward toning exercises or weights? Free weights or fixed weights? Fixed weights or Nautilus? Isometric or Isotonic? Dynamic or static? Conditioning or stretching? New York stretching or Californian stretching? The sheer confusion of choice alone can bring on a sense of overwhelming inertia…

What is needed is a programme which will integrate these methods because each has something to offer, but not everything. Combining them leads to a more complete form of fitness than following any one to the exclusion of the rest. This 24-week programme has been designed to promote all-round fitness and to get you into your best shape ever, by introducing each of these fitness basics – posture in week 1, stretch in week 3, aerobics in week 8, weights in week 9 and so on.

To guard against the possible risks of injury or of overdoing it, the programme is graduated, starting very gently and getting increasingly demanding as you get fitter. It takes a full 6 months to get into shape, to transform a flabby, out-of-condition body into a lean, fit one. Try to take short-cuts or treat exercise as a race and you are heading for trouble. The exercise boom may have focused some healthy, and much-needed, attention on our state of fitness, or lack of it, but it has also doubled the queues of people seeking the services of doctors, physiotherapists and osteopaths for sprained knees, bad backs, torn tendons and other sports-related aches and pains. The headlong rush to get fit is always self-defeating. You've got to be able to walk again before you can run again.

Avoid being an exercise drop-out by going at a reasonable pace and by remembering that healthy exercise has much more to do with beating the sluggish uninspired part of yourself than it does with beating anyone else. Twinges of pain are warnings to be careful, not challenges to be overcome.

Although you will find that the particular exercise focus changes each week, a general emphasis on self-awareness runs throughout the programme. As you become fitter, so you also become more aware of how your body feels as it moves and, gradually, more attuned to what your own unique fitness needs are. By week 24 you will not only be fit, strong and supple but also self-confident in the knowledge that you are well able to take good care of yourself and to continue exercising in the way that is right for you. And that's what being really fit and healthy is all about…

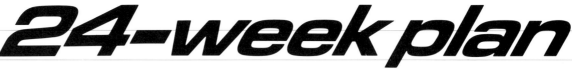

24-week plan

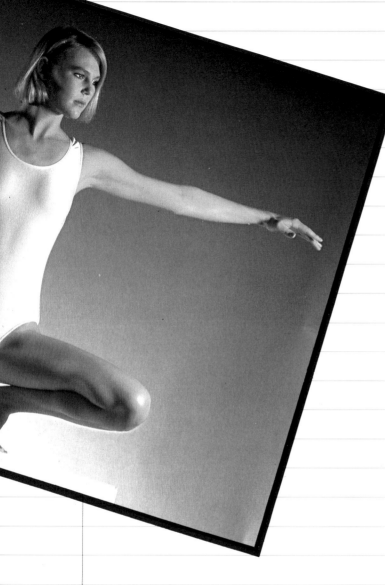

Follow the programme, starting today, from week one, repeating exercises as indicated on the lists at the beginning of each week. New exercises are underlined in black. Run through the programme every day if possible (and at least 3 times a week) at whatever time you like – but never directly after a heavy meal. Try to establish a regular exercise time because you will find it easier to stick to your programme if it becomes a normal part of your day. Wear clothes that are comfortable and which allow freedom of movement. Leotard, tracksuit, vest and pants, and loose baggy T-shirt over tights are all good. If knees are weak, leg warmers can be very useful.

The colour of leotard in each illustration varies with the type of exercise according to the key below. When an exercise combines two or more elements, the leotard is striped.

stretch	co-ordination
loosener	relaxation
mobility	aerobics
tester	balance
strengthener	therapeutics

WEEK 1: POSTURE

Good posture comes first for two reasons: it determines your shape and ensures you are working the right muscles and joints, so getting the most from your exercises...

If you have been told good posture means 'tummy in, chest out, shoulders back', you have been told wrong, for good posture starts from the back, not the front, and is achieved by a natural lengthening of the spine. The spine largely determines your shape because it communicates with every part of the body via skull, shoulders, ribcage and pelvic girdle. If its position is right, everything from top of head to toes automatically comes into line.

These Preliminaries will help realign your body by returning your spine to its correct position. Sense what happens to your body as you do them and repeat them often through the day – not just when you exercise. Feel what it is like to stand correctly with spine lengthened, shoulders down, pelvis centered and weight balanced and enjoy the feeling of lift that flows through you as you lengthen upwards.

This week's programme
Preliminaries
1 × 2
2 × 4 each way twice
3 × 8 each side
4 × several
5 × 16
6 × 1
7 × 5 each level
8 × 4 each side
9 × 1 each side
10 × 3
11 × up to 8 each side
12 × 8
13 × 2 each leg
14 × 4
15 × several
16 × several
17 × 7 each way
18 × 1

PRELIMINARIES

I **HEAD AND NECK** *Stand sideways to a mirror and let head drop down. Now lengthen at back of neck as you lift back of head. Feel yourself growing taller. Notice how lifting from back of head lengthens top of spine. But don't cheat by poking chin out as this will shorten top of spine by increasing curve at back of neck. Drop shoulders down away from ears to allow top of spine to lengthen upwards.*

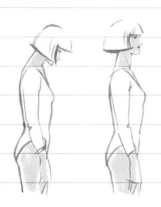

Maximum lengthening of the spine from coccyx to base of skull: good posture in a nutshell...

Posture is *the* instant shape-improver, much more effective than crash dieting. You can make your figure look 100 per cent better, *immediately*, by standing and moving correctly.

When posture is right, the bones and ligaments of the skeleton counteract the pull of gravity leaving muscles free for movement; when posture is wrong, muscles take over the work of the bones, producing unnecessary strains and tensions...

II PELVIS

Still standing sideways on to mirror, stick your bottom out and notice how this makes your tummy bulge too. See also how small of back has become more curved. Does this shortening of spine make the whole of your back feel tight? The correct position of spine is achieved by tilting pelvis into a central position. Place one hand on lower back, the other on tummy and gently push lower back forwards. Notice how small of back lengthens as pubic bone lifts a little and tummy is contained. This centering of pelvis is crucial to posture.

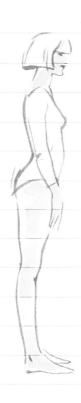

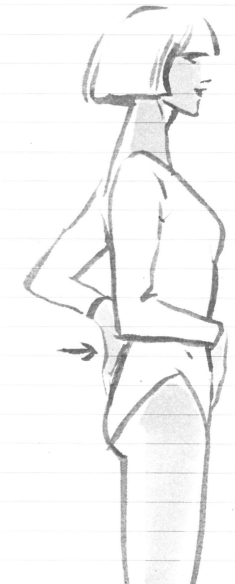

III WEIGHT BALANCE

Stand with legs slightly apart. How is your weight placed? Do you stand more on left side or right? Do you slightly bend one knee, placing all your weight on the other leg? Try doing this and notice what happens to your hips and shoulders. Now readjust posture so that hips and shoulders are level and you are standing with weight centrally balanced between heels and balls of feet.

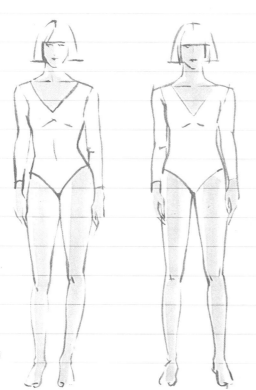

Once you have done them, run through Preliminaries again. Now you are ready to start exercising.

1 NECK *Stand correctly, remembering to lift at back of neck, and slowly lower head forwards as far as you can. Return it to centre and then, keeping lift in back of neck, lower it slowly backwards. Don't let it drop. Return head to centre and tilt it to right until you feel a gentle stretch along left side of neck, then bring it back to centre and repeat to left. Turn head to right, looking round as far as you can, then return to centre and repeat to left. Now repeat the exercise.*

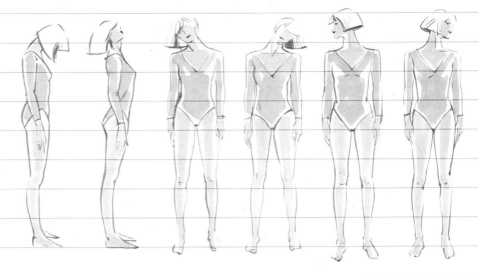

Ease into exercising with general stretches to lengthen muscles and prepare them for more strenuous work to come. Warmed extended muscles are more responsive to exercise, less susceptible to injury . . .

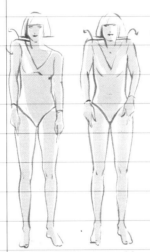

REMEMBER Drop shoulders and lengthen back of neck all the way through your exercise routine.

2 SHOULDERS *These loosen up the shoulder area, which is often stiff, and can be practised whenever you are aware of any tightness or tension there. Standing straight, take one shoulder forwards, lift it and then push it back and down. Repeat twice for each shoulder and then rotate them together 4 times, first forwards and then back. It is important to end on the backward movement as most people tend to let their shoulders come too far forwards.*

3 SIDES *Stand with feet apart and parallel. Raise both arms. Reach up further with alternate arms, feeling stretch at sides. Practise 8 times each side.*

4 UPPER BACK *Raise arms to shoulder level in front of you. Reach forwards with alternate arms and bring them back into place several times. Repeat with both arms together. Then try interlacing hands, turning palms away from you. Tuck buttocks underneath you and push away with hands, feeling stretch across back of shoulders.*

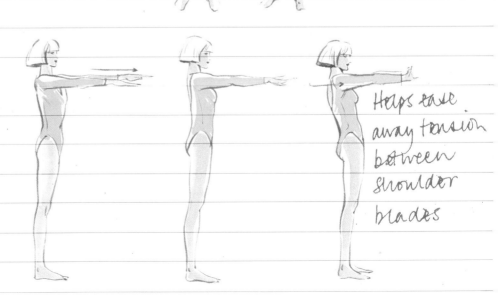

Helps ease away tension between shoulder blades

5 **LEGS** *Stand with feet slightly apart and parallel. Bend knees, keeping heels on floor. Straighten legs, lifting up onto balls of feet. Practise 16 times.*

CAUTION When bending knees, make sure they are directly above toes and do not fall inwards.

The weight of the head (over 4.5 kg/10 lb), the habit of holding it stiffly and the everyday effects of stress make for tense tight muscles that can lead to pain and headaches. This movement sequence will help loosen the muscles around the neck and so relieve strain.

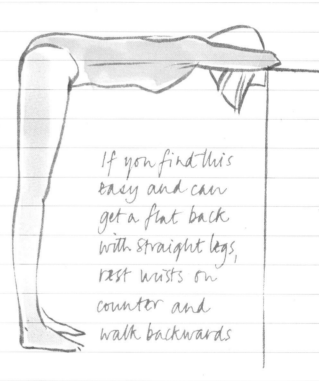

Strengthens legs and gets circulation going after standing still

6 **BACK** *This is an excellent exercise for beginners provided you are supported, so lower back is protected. Think about your posture as you do it and feel how helpful it can be for lengthening the back. Bend knees and bend forwards from hips, folding arms and resting elbows on a counter at about hip height. Walk backwards with knees slightly bent until you are making a right angle between trunk and legs. Now lengthen back of neck as you bend knees a bit more. Feel how this helps back to lengthen. Gradually straighten knees keeping length in back so it* remains as flat as possible. Repeat bending and straightening several times.

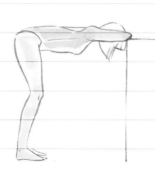

A strong stretch in the shoulders and arms may be felt at first as chest area expands.

If you find this easy and can get a flat back with straight legs, rest wrists on counter and walk backwards

7 **BUST** *Clasp hands in front of you and clench them sharply together 5 times at waist, shoulder and eye level in order to work every part of the supporting muscles.*

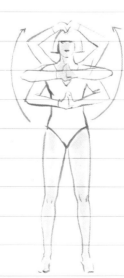

Strengthens muscles which help support the breasts

Muscle has just so much elasticity before it contracts back to its original shape. While slow easy stretching extends it according to these natural limits, quick bouncing movements do not. They should be avoided, or at least left till really fit, because they invoke the stretch reflex – which causes muscles to contract as a protective measure. Repetitive bouncing movements can cause damage to muscle and connective tissue because of the speed of the contraction, so keep stretches slow and controlled throughout the exercise programme.

8 WAIST *Stand with feet apart and slightly turned out. Lift ribs away from hips. Bend to side and hold for 3 counts, maintaining feeling of lift as you bend. Feel stretch along opposite side. Come back to centre and repeat to other side. Practise 4 times.*

Good posture is essential to get the most from this, so check you are standing well throughout.

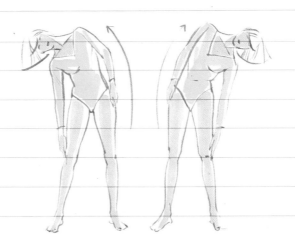

Imagine a pane of glass just behind and in front of you to prevent you tipping forwards or backwards

If your posture is perfect, your abdominal muscles will act like a belt to hold in your tummy. If you slouch, they will weaken and your tummy will stick out however slim you are.

Check posture by checking shoes. Where are the soles more worn down? If toes or heels, you are tipping too far forwards/ too far back when you walk; if outsides, you are rolling your feet outwards; if insides, weight is tipping inwards and knees are probably knocking together too.

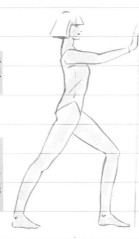

9 CALVES *Stand with one leg forwards and one back, heels firmly on floor, front knee bent and other straight with muscles at front of thigh contracted. Now lean forwards, using a wall for support if you find it helps, until you can feel a strong pull in calves. Maintain pull for 10 counts, and release. Change legs and repeat.*

10 BACKS OF THIGHS *Stand with feet a little apart and parallel. Bend knees as you bend forwards from hips, keeping back long. Slowly go down into a squat, so* *that front lower ribs are resting on about the middle of thighs. Allow heels to lift a little. Place hands on either side. Breathe in. As you breathe out, straighten legs as much as you can, but don't* *worry if you are unable to straighten knees. Feel stretch in backs of legs and continue to breathe out as you hold position for 4 counts. Breathe in as you squat down again. Practise 3 times.* *If you feel stretch behind knees, fine; if any pain in lower back, however, this exercise is not for you. Try mobility sequences for spine on page 122 and return to this when back becomes more mobile.*

THE AIM.... to keep ribs as close as possible to thighs as you straighten legs

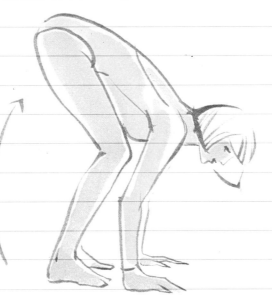

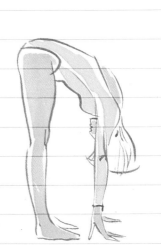

11 LUNGE *Stand well with feet together and arms out to side at shoulder level. Transfer weight from foot to foot, lifting heels and keeping toes on floor, several times. Then step from foot to foot, lifting feet about 20 cm (8 ins) from floor each time.*

When you feel well balanced, try this gentle aerobic exercise. Take one leg forwards, bending knee until it is directly over toes, and the other back so that you are now in a lunge position. Bend back knee and lift leg up in front of you. Replace it on floor behind. Practise up to 8 times and then change legs.

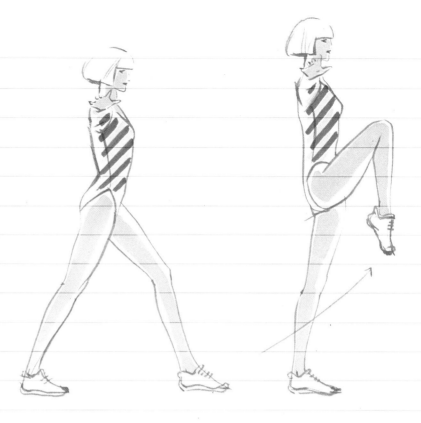

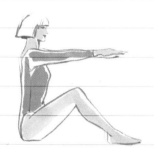

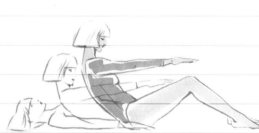

Feel tummy muscles working strongly

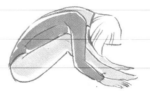

12 ABDOMEN *Sit on floor with knees bent; feet hip-width apart and arms straight out in front at shoulder level. Breathe in. As you breathe out, lean back tilting pelvis and lowering head. Press lower back into floor. Breathe in and come up. Breathe out and flop gently forwards. Breathe in and come up. Practise 8 times, in a good smooth rhythm.*

13 OUTER THIGHS *Lie on back with arms at shoulder level. Raise left knee into chest and extend leg upwards, flexing foot. Pass it over right thigh onto floor, aiming to get foot as close to right hand as possible. Feel stretch in left thigh and hold for 4 counts, breathing out and trying to keep shoulder blades flat on floor. Now lift leg again and, bending knee as before, lower to floor. Repeat with right leg. Then complete exercise again.*

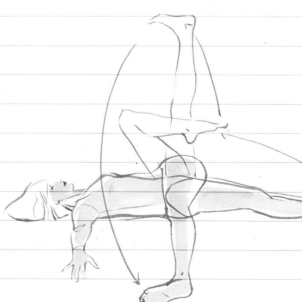

Bonus: Gives a marvellous twist in the spine

If aware of any strain in back, leave this one out and practise Therapeutic exercises on page 122 instead. Return to it when back gets stronger.

BONUS
Stretches
inner thighs
and loosens
hips.

14 *BACK* Sit with bottom against a wall and soles of feet together and as close to you as possible. Place hands on ankles and lengthen spine upwards so that shoulder blades and back of crown of head are touching wall too. Pull thighs downwards*, maintaining length in spine and hold for 4 counts. Practise 4 times.

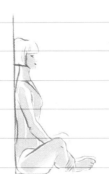

*Ask a friend to measure distance between knees and floor and note it down for reference later . . .

Used as a meditation pose for its excellent effects on posture and breathing. When spine is lengthened, ribs are lifted and chest opens, enabling you to breathe well.

CAUTION If you feel any pain in knees, bring feet away from you until comfortable.

15 *BACK* Now come away from wall and see if you can lengthen back upwards unsupported in another position. At first do this side-view to a mirror to check back is straight. Sitting, take legs apart until you feel a slight stretch in inner thighs. Now lengthen spine upwards as much as you can*. Look in mirror. Is back lengthened or rounded? If unable to straighten up completely, use hands to help. Place them behind you and push them into floor. Now hold position for a few moments and then round back and bend knees. Repeat several times, gradually increasing holding time to a minute or more.

As stretch in inner thighs subsides and you feel you can take more, push on hands, lifting trunk off floor a little; then lower a little further forwards so legs go further apart.

*How far can you comfortably take legs apart while maintaining length in spine? Ask a friend to measure distance between feet and note it down for reference later . . .

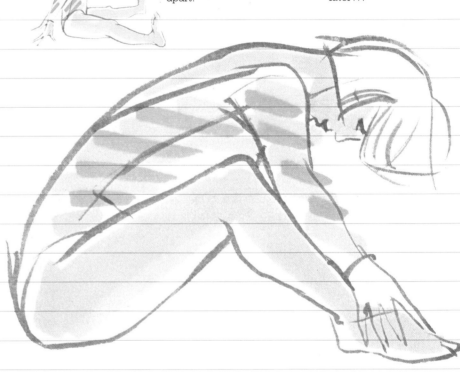

Releases tension in back and makes a good loosener after the strong posture exercises.

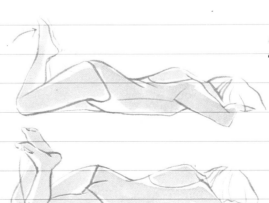

16 *BACK* Lie on front, hands flat one on top of the other and forehead on hands. Bend knees and let feet sway to each side several times.

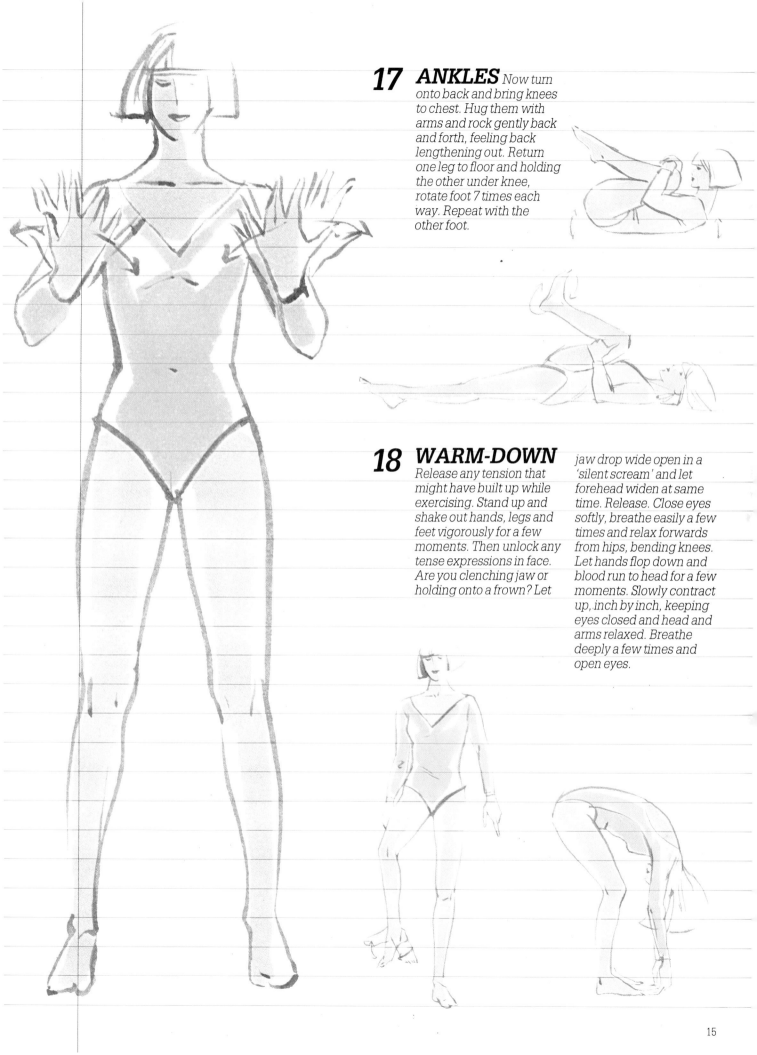

17 ANKLES *Now turn onto back and bring knees to chest. Hug them with arms and rock gently back and forth, feeling back lengthening out. Return one leg to floor and holding the other under knee, rotate foot 7 times each way. Repeat with the other foot.*

18 WARM-DOWN
Release any tension that might have built up while exercising. Stand up and shake out hands, legs and feet vigorously for a few moments. Then unlock any tense expressions in face. Are you clenching jaw or holding onto a frown? Let jaw drop wide open in a 'silent scream' and let forehead widen at same time. Release. Close eyes softly, breathe easily a few times and relax forwards from hips, bending knees. Let hands flop down and blood run to head for a few moments. Slowly contract up, inch by inch, keeping eyes closed and head and arms relaxed. Breathe deeply a few times and open eyes.

WEEK 2: BREATHING

Good breathing is the secret of successful exercising, enabling you to work to the best of your abilities and having considerable benefits for heart and health.

Although none of us needs to learn how to breathe any more than we need to learn how to make the heart beat, we do need to *relearn* how to use the whole of our breathing apparatus – namely the 12 pairs of ribs, and their intercostal muscles, that attach to either side of the spine and come round to form the sides and front of the chest.

To use your ribcage correctly, your posture must also be correct. If not, all the breathing exercises in the world will be to no avail for it is only when the spine is lengthened and chest lifted that the ribcage has the freedom it needs.

This week's programme
Preliminaries
14, see note, × 4
19 × 1
20 × several
6, with pelvic tilts
21 × several
22 × several
23 × 3 each side
24 × 1
25 × 8
26
27 × up to 12 each leg
12 × 8
13 × 2 each leg
28 × 4
15, progression **29** × 4
16 × several
30 × 7 each way
31

19 GOOD BREATHING

Now move away from wall and stand up, maintaining length in back and openness in chest. Place one hand on chest and the other on abdomen. Take a few slow deep breaths. Which hand moves first? If it is the upper one, you are breathing from the top of your chest, hardly using ribcage at all. Now continue breathing slowly and evenly, but concentrate on taking each breath down to bottom of ribs. Can you feel abdomen moving gently out as chest fills with air and the diaphragm, an involuntary muscle, moves downwards? Continue breathing in this way several times and then place hands across middle of back. Notice ribs are working there too. Breathing uses whole of the chest area, not just the front.

N.B. Back strengthener (**14**) will be familiar. Notice that your spine is not flattened against the wall but curves slightly in at the small of your back – just enough to get your hand through. This natural curve is good, if not too exaggerated, because it helps your chest to open and your ribs to work freely.

Now slump your shoulders forwards and notice what happens to your ribcage. See what happens, too, when you stiffen up and flatten your chest.

Returning to the correct position, become aware of your breathing. See how easy it is when you give yourself enough room.

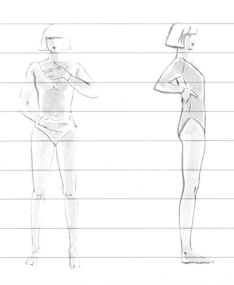

Few of us realize the extent of the breathing space available to us. We never think of our lungs expanding at the back as well as the front, for example.

20 **NECK** *Here is a progression of the exercise practised last week. Breathe in as you turn head to side. Breathing out, lower head slowly forwards and then breathe in again as you lift it to other side. Practise several times.*

Close eyes so you can attend fully to movement of ribs as you breathe

Breathe in through the nose as you prepare for the exercise, out through nose or mouth as you do it, and in again through the nose as you release. Instructions are given to help you. Don't worry if you feel like breathing in when the instructions say out. This often happens to begin with, particularly if you usually hold your breath when you exercise. Help counteract it by reminding yourself to BREATHE OUT. The out-breath is always the important one; the in-breath will look after itself.

21 **BACK** *Here is a progression on last week's flat back exercise (6). Start as before and go into flat back, resting elbows on counter for support. Now do a few pelvic tilts as you stand with knees straightened and back supported. Breathe in. As you breathe out, tilt pelvis, contracting tummy muscles and allowing back to round. Breathe in as you flatten back again. Practise several times.*

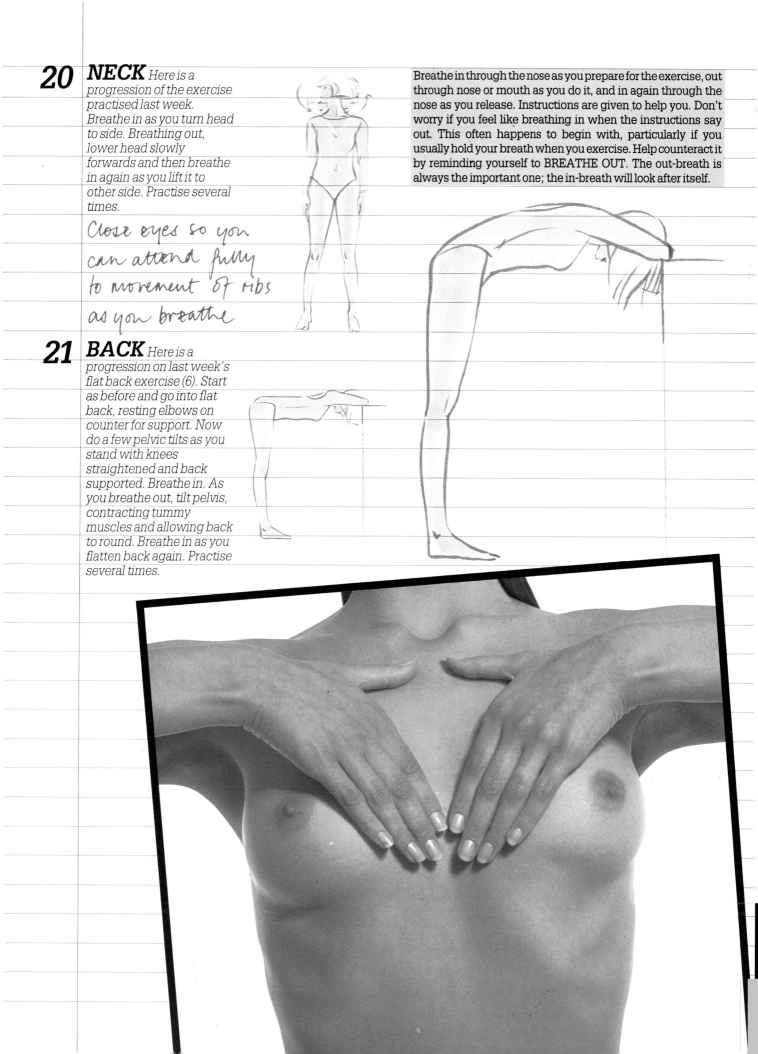

22 LOOSENER

Start by standing well, feet hip-width apart. Breathe in. As you breathe out, contract in and curl forwards, bending knees and allowing arms to flop forwards. Breathe in as you straighten knees. Enjoy it several times, moving easily and freely.

Notice you breathe out as front of body contracts, in as it expands: this is the principle behind all breathing when exercising.

Remember your good posture throughout

It is vital to breathe out properly. 70 per cent of all the body's waste is expelled on the breath. Compare with defecation (3 per cent), urination (7 per cent) and sweating (20 per cent) and you will see that in order to eliminate waste, and keep body tissues healthy and uncongested, it behoves us to breathe fully and freely. Vigorous sustained aerobic exercise will help to do this by giving lungs a good workout.

23 WAIST

This is a progression from last week's stretch (8). Stand with feet apart and parallel. Breathe in as you lift left arm (keeping shoulder pulled down). Breathe out as you bend to right, stretching as far as you can. Breathe in as you come up a little, allowing arm to bend. Breathe out as you stretch again to side. Repeat twice and then change arms.

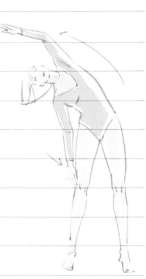

Use your breathing to help you when you exercise – a long exhale can help you stretch a bit further or contract your muscles more strongly . . .

24 CHEST AND BACKS OF THIGHS

Stand with feet apart. Breathe in and take hands behind, clasping them together. As you breathe out, lift hands up as far as possible and bend forwards from hips. Breathe normally as you hold stretch for 4 counts, then hold it for a further 4 taking good deep breaths and feeling reaction in abdomen. Shake head gently to make sure neck muscles feel free. Breathe in and straighten.

Excellent for posture

If you can't yet bend from hips with flat back, bend knees as you go forwards.

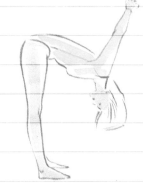

25 LEGS

A progression on last week's strengthener (5). This time, take legs wider apart and point feet out so that legs turn out from hip joint and knees are aligned over toes. Place hands on hips to help keep pelvis centered. Breathe in as you straighten legs and lift heels. Practise 8 times.

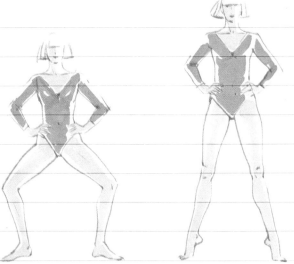

26 UPPER BODY

This excellent exercise encourages good breathing, strengthens chest, bust and arms and gives a stretch along backs of legs. Stand arm's length away from a wall with feet together and arms at shoulder level. Place palms flat on wall in front. Breathe in. As you breathe out, bend arms and lean forwards, keeping spine in a long straight line. Breathe in as you return to starting position. Practise 4 press-ups, rest a moment, and repeat.

As exercise gets easier, step back further

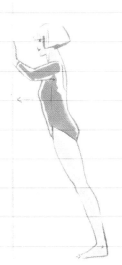

27 KICK

Try this progression of last week's aerobic exercise (11), keeping lunge position but instead of bending knee and lifting leg, kick it out in front. Practise up to 12 kicks each leg.

Place your hands on your chest after doing the leg kicks. If not actually panting, you will certainly be breathing rapidly and from the top of your chest. Next time you feel tense or anxious, examine your breathing again. Are you breathing too fast and too high? Take slower, deeper breaths and feel yourself relax...

28 ABDOMEN

Lie flat on back with body in a long straight line, shoulders down and arms at sides. Bend knees, so that feet are flat on floor, hip-width apart. Breathe in. As you breathe out, lift head and shoulders off floor. Hold for 3 counts if you can. Breathe in as you lower to floor. Practise 4 times* and then roll head from side to side to release front neck muscles (they have to work strongly in this exercise). Take a good deep breath to release any tension in chest too.

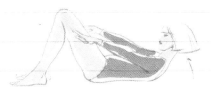

If you feel strain in neck, place one or two cushions under head.

*Next time you try this, see how many you can do comfortably, *without straining*. It may be no more than 4 or 5. Note it down for reference later...

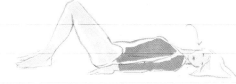

It is important to get your breathing right on the strong abdominal exercises (12 and 28) because the chest on the in-breath is like a full balloon: the intake of air builds up pressure, pushing the tummy out. It is physiologically impossible, therefore, to contract it at the same time. It is by breathing out that you work these muscles...

29 BACK

Try this active progression of last week's back strengthener (15). Starting as before, sitting on floor with legs well apart and spine lifted, hold for as long as you can breathing normally. Then breathe in, lifting spine a little more. Now interlace fingers, take palms away from you and, as you breathe out, do a pelvic tilt allowing back to round and knees to bend, pushing forwards with hands. Breathe in straightening legs strongly and lifting back. Coordinating movements with breathing should produce a nice steady rhythm. Practise 4 times. Bring legs together and shake them out to release any tension after this strong exercise.

BONUS Gives a good stretch across back

Do you feel like yawning when you exercise? If so, it is a good sign because it is the body's natural way of getting more air and means you are working muscles well, increasing their demand for oxygen.

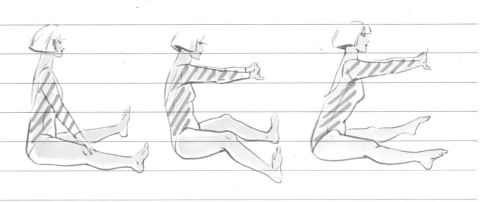

Your breathing not only reflects every physical effort but every emotional disturbance too. When angry, your breathing becomes shallow and quick; when excited, you take longer out-breaths, breathe in more quickly; when depressed, you continue to take air in and let hardly any out. When very strongly moved or surprised, you (momentarily) stop breathing altogether...

30 ANKLES AND WRISTS

Now turn onto back and press knees into chest. Hold arms loosely in air, as shown, and then rotate feet and hands together, 7 times each way.

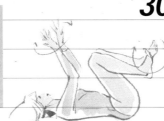

31 RELAXATION

Still lying on back, slide feet down along floor. Bring them together and flex feet as you lift head to look between them. Now lower head and allow legs to rotate easily outwards. Turn palms of hands upwards so arms rotate outwards too. Take 3 or 4 good deep breaths thinking about using ribcage to its maximum so that it lifts up and out on

in-breath and sinks back on out-breath. It may help to imagine you are lying by the sea: with each in-breath waves wash over you and with each out-breath they race back to the ocean. Stay there for a while, with eyes closed. Notice how breathing becomes shallower and more even as body quietens and needs less and less oxygen to keep it going.

Looking down midline of body helps you to check that you are lying in a straight line

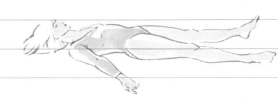

WEEK 3: STRETCH

Good breathing can be applied very successfully to long, slow stretching – the essential preliminary to any activity whether it is jogging, yoga, aerobics, weight training or simply getting out of bed in the morning...

The gentle stretches you have been doing will have helped lengthen your muscles in preparation for this week's stronger ones. As you do them, you may find strong resistance in parts of your body. This is an uncomfortable sensation – not pain (*see note, over*) – and it will make your body want to tighten up to protect itself. Help prevent this natural tendency by breathing OUT as you work through the stretch and you will find that the sensation subsides, enabling you to stretch still further.

This week's programme
Preliminaries
32 × several
3 × several
33 × 6 backwards
34 × 8 each side
35 × 8 each leg
27 × 8 each side
36 × 8 each side
6, progression **37** × 4
25 × 8
26, taking feet further from wall × 8
24, trying to straighten legs × 1
12 × 4
28, taking head, shoulders and ribs off floor × 4
13 × 3 each leg
30 × 7 each way
29 × 4
38 × 1 each leg
39 × 1
31

Listen to your body and be aware of its needs. If stiff or tense at the start of your session, spend longer than usual on the stretches until you feel really loosened up. Swinging straight into a demanding routine will otherwise merely be adding to tensions that are already there...

32 **WARM-UP** *Stand well, with feet hip-width apart and parallel. Breathe in and stretch up as you lift arms. Breathe out as you bend knees and swing down. Straighten knees a little before bending them to help you swing up again on an in-breath. Enjoy this warm-up several times and then continue with small upwards stretches as though climbing a rope-ladder to ceiling.*

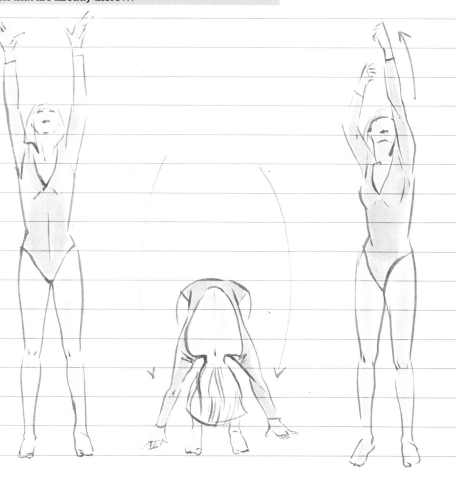

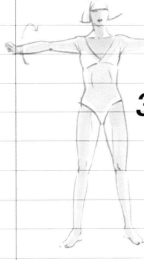

33 SHOULDERS

Lower arms sideways to shoulder level, turning feet out a little so that legs rotate from hips. Now make 6 small backward circles with arms, feeling a good stretch across front of chest each time.

Stretching, and particularly regular stretching, brings all sorts of benefits: greater flexibility, more freedom from tension, less likelihood of stiffness or physical injury, a strong sense of mental and physical well-being. Hold each stretch for count of 8, then, if comfortable, for a further 8 for extra lengthening – breathing well throughout.

IMPORTANT Learn to distinguish between the good stretch feeling of the well-used muscle and pain, which is more acute and actually *hurts*. Exercise should never hurt. If pain is felt, stop at once and consult your doctor.

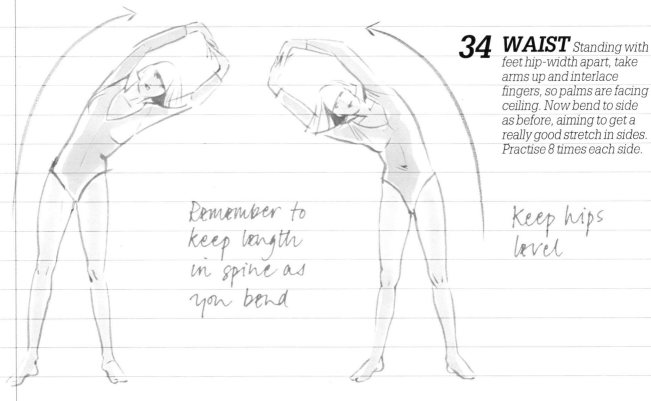

34 WAIST
Standing with feet hip-width apart, take arms up and interlace fingers, so palms are facing ceiling. Now bend to side as before, aiming to get a really good stretch in sides. Practise 8 times each side.

Remember to keep length in spine as you bend

Keep hips level

If you find that you can stretch further on one side than the other, give the stiffer side a chance to catch up by working it a little more and adding a few more repetitions.

Aim for same looseness in hips when walking

35 HIPS
Stand well with spine lifted, holding onto wall or back of chair for support. Now raise outside arm to shoulder level and swing leg forwards and back loosely from hip joint 8 times. Change legs and repeat.

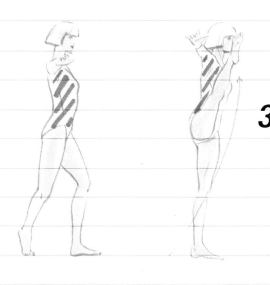

Stiffness not only restricts movement, it restricts pleasure too. Stretching can help bring more joy and spontaneity to your lovemaking by making you more supple, more sensuous, more confident in and about your body...

36 KICK *Stand with arms out sideways at shoulder level. Take one leg behind you and across, so that you are standing with weight on forward foot and toes of other foot resting on floor behind. Now breathe in and bend supporting leg a little. Breathe out as you kick to side with toes pointed. Practise 8 times, then change legs and repeat.*

37 BACK *Take legs wide apart and stand with feet parallel. Breathe in, raise arms to ceiling and stretch upwards. As you breathe out, go forwards from hips into flat back position. Continue on down till hands reach floor and stay there, breathing well, as you allow stretch to subside. Breathe in and lift. Breathe out and lower hands to floor again. Repeat 3 times to the rhythm of your breathing.*

If not much stretch is felt, walk hands backwards towards feet.

38 BACK AND LEGS *Sit on floor with back well lengthened. Breathe in and lengthen back a little more. As you breathe out, bend forwards from hips and hold flexed foot first with inside hand and then with both hands together. Breathe in and lift. As you breathe out, lower over extended leg. Hold for a few moments and, if stretch subsides, lengthen body down a little further. Repeat exercise with other leg, breathing well throughout. If you cannot reach feet with hands, use towel or belt round foot as illustrated on next exercise.*

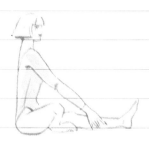
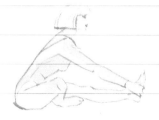

Eventually this becomes relaxing, particularly when you are loose enough at hips to rest head on legs. If you haven't yet found this, relax by stretching out as last week.

39 BACK AND LEGS *Now try forward bend with both legs straight and feet flexed. Use a towel or belt round feet at first, as shown here. Holding onto towel, breathe in and lift up. Maintaining length in your back, breathe out and bend forwards from hips. Creep hands further down towel and go as far as you can, keeping back quite straight*. Don't let it round. With practice you will soon hold outsides of feet.*

The body's response to stress is to stiffen up—shoulders tense, fists clench, expression freezes as blood races to the large muscle groups and the body armours itself for 'fight, flight or fright'. This primitive survival response can produce deeply-ingrained tensions that interfere with our zest and enjoyment of life. Using stretching and breathing to overcome internal tensions may help you manage external ones better...

*Now try this without a towel, looking in a mirror. How far can you go maintaining your flat back? Mark it with a dotted line on the diagram for progress reference later on...

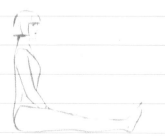

[handwritten margin notes] + very important stretch that lengthens hole of nck of body + legs

WEEK 4: AWARENESS

Exercising can increase awareness as long as each movement is sensed fully and not just repeated a set number of times. That is the message of Moshe Feldenkrais, Israeli physicist, teacher and philosopher, whose work has done so much to show how movement can be a path both to greater self-awareness and to unlocking hidden potential. 'Know what you are doing,' he says, 'and you can do what you want.'

This week's exercises 40-45 are based on his work. They are not 'exercises' in the traditional sense – not being designed to lose inches or strengthen muscles – but to increase awareness by freeing you from habit, and guiding you towards new ways of moving. New ways of moving can ultimately become new ways of being, because freeing the body enables the mind to develop freely too. Do the exercises slowly, concentrating on every stage, to help sharpen awareness.

This week's programme

Preliminaries
40 × several
41 × several
42 × several
43 × several
44 × 40 each side
45 × several
39, or with one leg bent if difficult **38**, × 1
13 × 4 each leg
34 × 8 each side
46 × 8 each leg
27 × 8 each leg
36 × 8 each leg
47 until comfortably out of breath
Active recovery cool-down, see page 41
37 × 6
26 until muscles being to tire
12 × 4
28 until muscles begin to tire
18 × 1
41 × several
31

---

40 **HABITS** *Interlace fingers together several times. Notice which thumb is on top and which little finger on the bottom. Is it always the same? Now repeat movement, but this time interlace fingers in non-habitual way so other thumb is on top. Does it feel strange and 'wrong'? Try it several times. Now do the same thing with your arms and then legs – crossing them first in the way that feels most natural and then doing the opposite. These movements are all habits and, though apparently unimportant, indicative of other habits that restrict and limit us.*

Until muscles begin to tire means stopping the exercise at the point where the muscles feel well-used, even capable of more, but where you feel no longer fresh enough to continue to do the exercise correctly. Too few repetitions are better than too many…

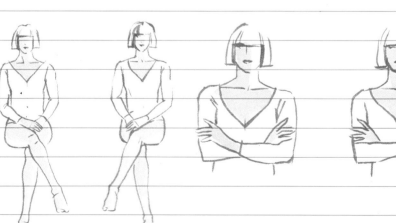

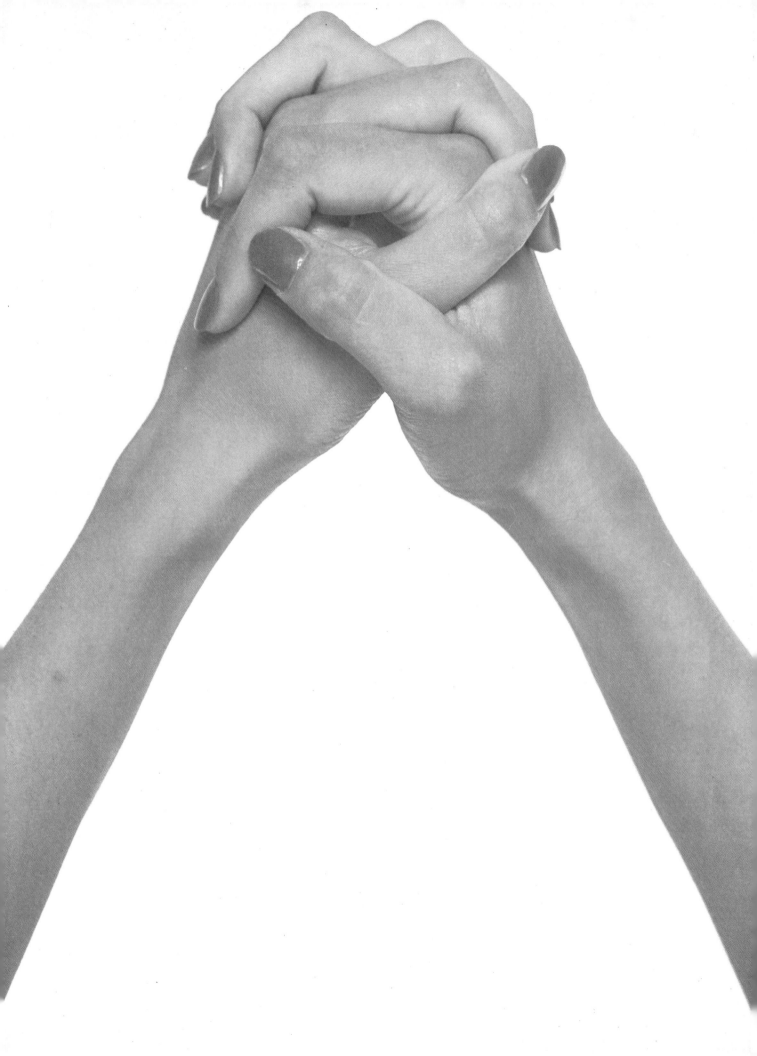

41 SPINE, HIPS, SHOULDERS

Lie on back with knees bent and feet flat on floor, about 15 to 20 cm (6 to 8 ins) apart. Arms, head, knees and shoulders should all be soft and relaxed. Notice what happens to your breathing as you try these movement combinations. Start by lifting one shoulder off floor several times and setting it back down. Repeat with other shoulder. Then with one hip and again with the other. Slide knees to floor and take a rest. Raise knees again and try lifting one shoulder and its opposite hip several times. Repeat with other shoulder and hip. Now lift both shoulders together several times and follow with both hips. Slide knees to floor and rest a moment. Raise knees again and lift one shoulder and hip on the same side together several times. Repeat with other shoulder and hip. Slide knees down and rest a moment and then try all the combinations again. Do they feel any easier?

'There is an essential difference between consciousness and awareness, although the borders are not clear in our use of language. I can walk up the stairs of my house, fully conscious of what I am doing, and yet not know how many steps I have climbed. In order to know how many there are I must climb them a second time, pay attention, listen to myself, and count them. Awareness is consciousness together with a realization of what is happening within it or of what is going on within ourselves while we are conscious.'
Moshe Feldenkrais

Vary your way of moving each time, sensing the differences for yourself. Start very slowly, seeing how long you can take to make a movement, and then try it more quickly; practise making very large exaggerated movements then tiny ones – the smallest you can make.

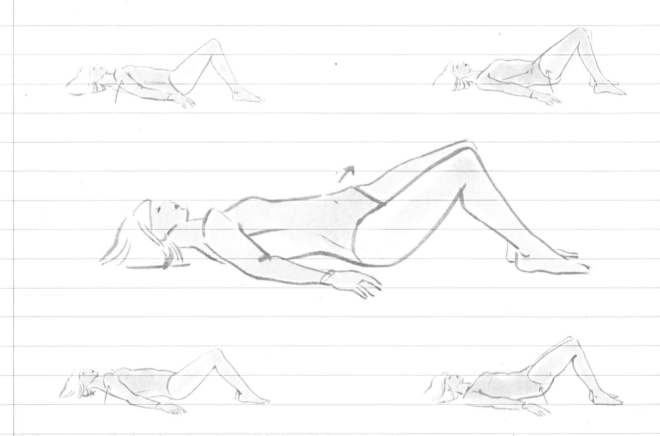

Do the sequences slowly and gently, and you will find your body gains quickly in agility as you gain in awareness. Differences can often be felt after just a few minutes. In addition bear the following in mind:

1. DON'T PUSH THROUGH PAIN. Each movement should be easy and fluid.

2. SLOW IS BETTER THAN FAST. Swift movements and mindless repetition reinforce habit; slow movements let you find new ways of moving. If aware of any stiffness or pain, slow down even more, so you can learn how to move without pain.

3. THE MEANS IS MORE IMPORTANT THAN THE END. Having a goal in mind limits you from the start because you shut off alternative possibilities. Keep an open mind, attend simply to each movement as you do it, pausing at each stage, and you will soon become aware of all the choices open to you and so will be able to pick the one that works best...

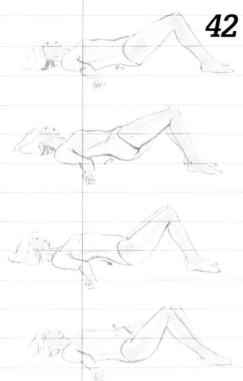

42 PELVIS

Lie on back and raise knees with legs in line with pelvis, hands by side and feet resting flat on floor. Imagine there is a clock face on the back of your pelvis, with 6 o'clock beneath coccyx and 12 o'clock just below navel. Move pelvis to 12 o'clock and notice that lower back lies flat on floor. Move between 6 and 12 o'clock slowly a number of times, being aware of how you organize this simple movement in your pelvic region.

Now imagine 3 o'clock beneath left hip and 9 o'clock beneath right hip. Rock slowly from side to side 20 times feeling both points. Rest a moment. Now move from 1 to 7 back and forth across face of pelvic clock; from 10 to 4; from 2 to 8; from 5 to 11 all several times.

Try this sequence: 12 to 1; 1 to 12; 12 to 11; 11 to 12 to 1; 1 to 12 to 11 to 10; 10 to 11 to 12 to 1 to 2; 2 to 1 to 12; 12 to 1 to 2 to 3; 3 to 2 to 1 to 12 to 11; 11 to 12 to 1 to 2 to 3; 3 to 2 to 1 to 12 to 11; 11 to 12 to 1 to 2 to 3; 3 to 2 to 1 to 12 to 11 to 10; 10 to 11 to 12 to 1 to 2; 2 to 1 to 12 to 11 to 10 to 9; 9 to 10 to 11 to 12. Stop and rest. Was there any area, say from 9 to 11, which was difficult or painful? Return to that area and move back and forth through it until movement becomes easier. Rest again. Now return to 6 to 12 movement. Is it any easier? Are you beginning to reclaim awareness of your pelvis? Rest a moment.

Now move to the 6 position. Move from 6 to 7; 7 to 6 to 5; 5 to 6 to 7; 7 to 6 to 5 to 4; 4 to 5 to 6 to 7; 7 to 6 to 5 to 4 to 3; 3 to 4 to 5 to 6 to 7 to 8; 8 to 7 to 6 to 5; 5 to 6 to 7 to 8 to 9; 9 to 8 to 7 to 6; 6 to 7 to 8 to 9 to 10 to 11 to 12. Stop and rest a moment. Then return to the 12 position and continue around face of clock in a clockwise direction, slowly taking 30 seconds to a minute for one rotation. Imagine you are the second hand making a sweep of the clock face. Repeat it several times. Stop and rest. Then make anti-clockwise circuits equally slowly. Stop and rest.

Your pelvis is your centre of gravity, sexuality and energy ... You have probably not moved it fully in years. Enjoy the pelvic clock movements, letting your energy flow freely. Isn't your pelvis more responsive, more supple than you imagined it could be? What other areas have you ceased to be aware of in this way?

BONUS
Gives the
spine a
good twist

43 UPPER BACK

Lie on back with feet flat on floor, 30 to 45 cm (12 to 18 ins) from buttocks, and knees bent vertically above them. Now raise both arms towards ceiling and place palms of hands together, so that armpits and wrists make angles of a triangle. Let arms fall to one side several times, keeping elbows straight and palms together. Don't let triangle collapse or you lose benefit of exercise. Feel opposite shoulder pushing arms over and notice how neck tends to lift from floor as arms move downwards. Repeat movement until you begin to notice arms tiring. Stop and rest. Then repeat again several times. Rest. Repeat.

44 LOWER BACK

Lying as before, but with arms by side, place right leg over left. Let both knees fall to right, keeping shoulder blades on floor. Both legs should now be supported by left foot only. Feel weight of right leg pulling left one down to floor and notice that when knees move down to floor neck tends to move away from floor. Return knees to centre and notice that neck returns to floor. Practise 20 times breathing out as you move knees downwards, in as you return them to central position. Stop and rest a moment and then repeat 20 times again. This time become aware of twist in spine and lengthening of muscles at side of vertebrae. Now stop and rest again and then reverse position, so that left leg is crossed over right. Let your knees fall to left 20 times, being aware of your body again, then rest a moment and repeat. Which side is more supple?

CAUTION Gives powerful twist in lower back. If you have back problems do it very gently, stop if you feel any pain and try Feldenkrais mobility sequences in Therapeutics section instead.

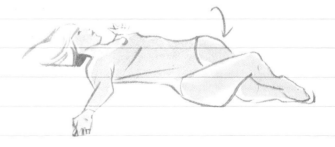

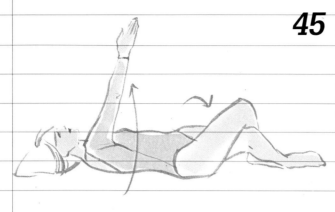

45 BACK *Now combine the last 2 exercises, letting hands and knees fall to opposite sides. Do this very gently and slowly, being aware of strong twist in spine. Do not force movement. Repeat several times. Then change way legs are crossed, let your knees fall to other side and take your arms over in opposite direction.*

Remember to keep elbows straight

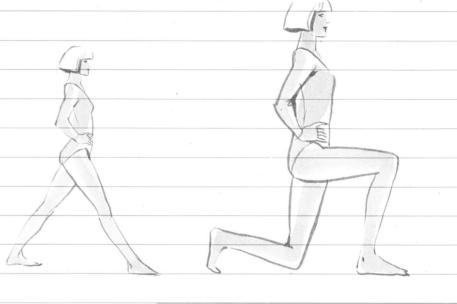

46 LEGS *Stand well with feet together. Take a large stride forwards with one foot, so that hips and feet are facing straight ahead. Do a small pelvic tilt and maintain it throughout. Breathe in. As you breathe out, bend front leg and lower back knee until it is touching (not resting on) floor. Return to starting position and repeat 7 times. Then repeat exercise with other foot in front.*

Good warm-up before running

Comfortably out of breath means stopping the exercise at a point well *before* breathlessness. You should be able to speak or to count yourself through the exercise while maintaining good technique for it to continue to have aerobic benefits. Once you start panting and gasping for air, the exercise has ceased to be aerobic and is no longer beneficial.

47 RUN *Running on the spot can be an excellent aerobic exercise but it needs a gradual build-up. Start simply by transferring weight from foot to foot, lifting heels only. Continue by lifting and stretching each foot. Then start to jump lightly from foot to foot so you are 'jogging' with feet about 10 cm (4 ins) off floor. Make sure you use whole of foot as you run – not just the balls. Gradually lift legs higher and continue until comfortably out of breath. Work down in same way afterwards to allow heart rate to slow.*

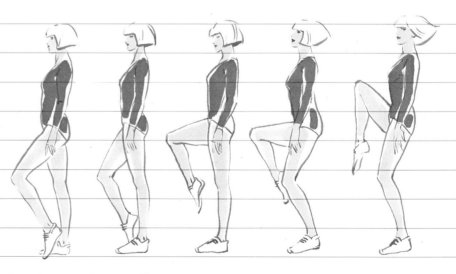

See also notes on running, page 98.

28

WEEK 5: TWISTS

Maintaining mobility in the spine is your key to a strong healthy back. The stiffness that leads to back problems in later life is often caused by loss of mobility: 'If you don't move it,' the saying goes, 'you lose it'.

Vertebrae are actually designed to move and it's through rotating and twisting exercises that move the spine laterally, as well as forwards and back, that they are kept supple. But twists must be done correctly for best benefit. Remembering your good posture, always lengthen well first so that each vertebra has room to move and is not compressed on top of the other.

To begin with, you may find that you don't feel much of a twist at all – the vertebrae may feel locked and the whole spine stiff. But persevere and you will find that you can go round a little further each time. Your spine will soon become more supple with practice.

This week's programme

Preliminaries
32 × several
STRETCHES (fill in exercises on lines provided)
....

48 × 3
49 × several
46 × 8 each leg
AEROBICS until comfortably out of breath
....

ABDOMEN STRENGTHENERS until muscles begin to tire
....

51 × 1 each side
BACK STRENGTHENER
....

43, 44, 45 × several
39, or with one leg bent **38**, × 1
52 × several
WARM-DOWN/ RELAXATION

Sense which ways of moving work best for you and make the most of this information by creating your own exercise routine. This week's basic structure ensures you work out in a sensible order (*see note*); the rest is up to you. Fill in with exercises from previous week that you found helpful, changing the routine each time.

NB When exercising it's not just what you do that's important, it's the order in which you do it. Warm up first with general stretches; follow with twists and looseners; aerobics to get heart and lungs going; then strengtheners and more advanced stretches, finishing with at least 10 minutes relaxation...

---

hank off where hands are on stick and bring them in as shoulders become more supple

48 CHEST *Stand well with pelvis centered, feet hip-width apart. Take a light broom or broomstick and hold it so your hands are about 1.2 m (4 ft) apart. Breathe in. As you breathe out, lift stick up, back and down as far behind you as you can. Breathe in. Breathe out and reverse process. If you find this very easy, bring hands further in until you can feel a good stretch across front and a contraction, or squeezing, in upper back. If it's very hard, take hands a little further out. Practise 3 times.*

49 **WAIST AND BACK** *Place stick across shoulders as shown. Stand with legs hip-width apart, feet parallel and knees bent over toes. Check pelvis is centered. Breathe in. As you breathe out, twist to one side turning head and eyes too. Breathe in as you return to centre. Breathe out as you twist to other side. Repeat several times in a good slow rhythm, spotting something behind you each time to prevent dizziness.*

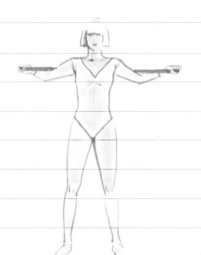
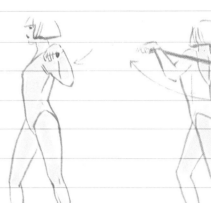

keep hips facing forward as much as possible for maximum twist in back

BONUS Stick helps you twist further because when shoulders are kept still, ribs are lifted and back is lengthened.

How many repetitions are right for you? Bear in mind it's not just practice, but *perfect* practice, that makes perfect. Once you get tired or sloppy, you start practising your own mistakes – so reinforcing them. Stop at the point where you *begin* to feel too tired to do the exercise correctly.

Did you find last week's way of working beneficial? Has it helped with your stretches, made you feel looser, more 'at home' in your body? If so, always include some Feldenkrais work when you exercise …

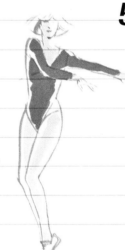

50 **JUMPS** *Prepare for this by standing with feet hip-width apart. Bend knees as you take arms over to one side, then straighten legs and lift heels from floor as you raise arms up to ceiling. Bend knees again and take arms to opposite side. Repeat 8 times, then start jumping lightly with both feet together, twisting body from side to side. Let arms swing freely in opposite direction. Continue until comfortably out of breath.*

51 **WAIST** *Sitting cross-legged on floor, feel two 'sitting' bones beneath you as you lengthen spine upwards and drop shoulders down. Place one hand across body onto opposite knee and take free hand onto floor behind. Breathe in and push down onto hand to lengthen spine a little more. Breathe out as you twist, pulling gently further round as you are able. Repeat to other side. Cross legs other (non-habitual) way and repeat.*

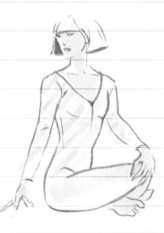

52 **BACK** *Lie on back with legs bent up, arms out at shoulder level and palms flat on the floor. Keeping knees together, take legs to one side and head to other. Keep shoulder blades on floor throughout. Repeat several times in an easy rhythm.*

BONUS Excellent tension releaser

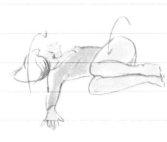

Are you becoming aware of some of the benefits of regular exercise? Do you feel stronger, supple, more self-aware and in tune with your body? Are you beginning to understand its needs?

Although you should feel well-used after exercising, you should not feel exhausted – rather alert, refreshed and ready for more. If you are not yet finding this, a good massage can often help because it gives that sensation of feeling calm yet energized at the same time …

WEEK 6: RELAXATION

It may seem odd to include a week on relaxation in a programme about movement, but the ability to relax is one of the most important elements of fitness. It is no use being strong and agile if you cannot relax because it is the balance between the two that produces real health.

Tension is tiring and wasteful – the inner result of outer pressures and problems that are often beyond your control. Help must therefore be sought from within. Finding inner resources that you can use to release muscular tension and to calm the mind is what learning to relax is about. For, although we all have these resources, we need to be taught how to apply them.

This week's programme

Preliminaries
32 × several
3 × several
53 × several
34 × 8 each side
46 × 8 each leg
47 until comfortably out of breath
54 until comfortably out of breath
Active recovery cool-down, see page 41
37 × 6
26 until muscles begin to tire
24 × 1
28 until muscles begin to tire
52 × several
55 × several
44 × 40 each side
39, or with one leg bent **38,** × 1
56 × 1
57 × 3 mins each foot
56 × 1
58

53 WARM-UP *A*
progression on last week's exercise with the broomstick. Stand with arms at shoulder level and swing around bending knee and lifting heel as you go. Focus on something on a wall behind to help prevent dizziness. Repeat to other side and continue twisting from side to side in a good easy rhythm until you feel really warmed up.

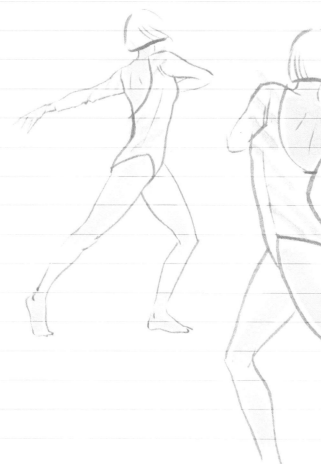

Tension exhausts mind as well as body. A brain buzzing with problems and preoccupations soon loses its creativity – its ability to find new solutions and to come up with fresh ideas. Freedom from anxiety requires a greater mental freedom and that can only happen when the mind is calm.

31

There are many different routes to relaxation and they don't all require you to be still. In fact, activity can be one of the best. Slow progressive stretching helps release tense contracted muscles while a more vigorous work-out can promote tremendous physical and mental calm.

54 JUMP KICK
Standing with both feet together, hop onto one leg as you bring other up towards chest. Now jump both feet together again and extend same leg forwards in a kick. Repeat, alternating legs, until comfortably out of breath.

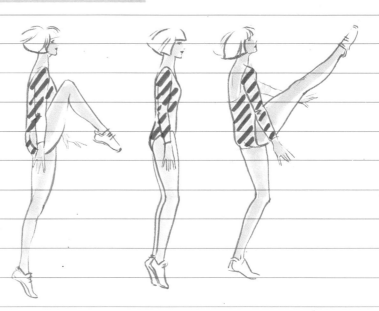

55 ABDOMEN
Lying on back with knees bent and feet flat on floor, breathe in. As you breathe out, push back of waist firmly into floor so pubic bone rises upwards. Pull tummy in at same time. Breathe in and release. Repeat several times.

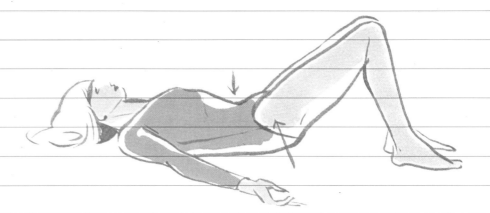

56 ROLL
Stand with feet hip-width apart and weight of body evenly distributed between them. Centre pelvis. Now lower head very slowly, tucking chin in. Continue lowering head towards floor and let shoulders drop forwards too, so arms are hanging heavily down. Bend knees as you go on curling VERY SLOWLY towards floor. Breathe well several times, then curl up again, equally slowly, keeping knees bent. Feel pelvis centering itself as you return equally slowly to upright position and straighten legs.

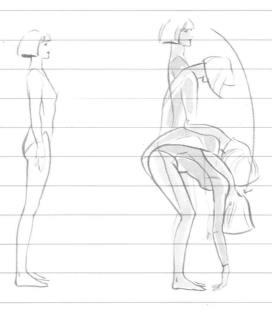

As you go down note tension points — places that feel difficult or stiff and interrupt flow of movement

57 FEET *Take a small firm ball – a squash ball is ideal – and place it beneath right foot. Roll it gently around in small circles, putting weight on foot. Imagine ball is covered with ink and you want to cover entire underside of foot – heel, sole, inner and outer edges, underneath toes. Continue for at least 3 minutes, closing eyes and enjoying massage.*

Now look at yourself carefully in a mirror. Is there a difference between the two sides of your body? Does right side feel more relaxed? Is right shoulder lower than left? If so, it is because massage has eased muscles on right side of body. Repeat *massage with other foot and see if, afterwards, both shoulders are level. Then repeat previous exercise and see if those areas of tightness have disappeared...*

Feet must be bare for this one

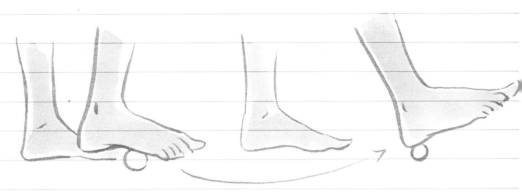

58 RELAXATION *Lie flat on back on floor. Press on elbows and back of head to raise chest a little, then pull shoulders away from ears. Lower chest again, spreading shoulder blades outwards and dropping chin slightly, so that back of neck is lengthened. Place one hand lightly on chest and other on abdomen and let* *them rest there. Rotate thighs outwards and wiggle knees until comfortable. This is your starting position.*

Now roll head from side to side to make sure any tension in neck is released. Press head down into floor and stop. Pull shoulders down away from body once more and stop. Tilt pelvis, pressing back of *waist into floor, and stop. Push heels away from you, lengthening backs of legs, and stop. Take a good deep breath, feeling lower hand rise as air is drawn deep into lungs. As you breathe out, release into floor and feel lower hand falling as air leaves lungs, but don't let your chest collapse. Run through your body checking for areas of* *tension. Are your jaws clenched? Are you frowning? Have shoulders crept up again? Is breathing still easy? Be aware of your body as you do this, then let go of everything, close eyes and relax, feeling breathing becoming shallower and shallower as you enter a state of deep relaxation.*

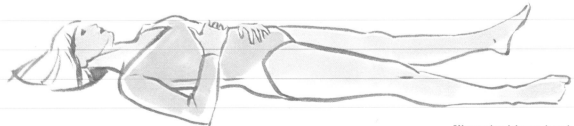

Ask someone to read this through as you do it

If lower back hurts, bend knees so feet are flat on floor, press lower back into floor until pain subsides, then slowly slide legs down again.

WEEK 7: STRENGTH

Building up strength may sound strenuous and difficult, but as soon as you begin you will discover that strength is about finding things easy. You will not feel so stiff after exercise; you will not get out of breath so soon; you will be able to manage everyday stresses and strains better and your posture and general shape will improve as your muscles become firmer and more toned. You should feel better too because while you are building up strength you will be giving your heart and lungs the boost they probably need.

As you work through your programme this week, be aware of what strengthening is all about. Sense your muscles tightening and contracting strongly as you exercise. Feel the warm tension and work them to the point where they begin to tire, but never continue until it becomes painful.

This week's programme

Preliminaries
32 × several
3 × several
53 × several
34 × 8 each side
59 × 16
47 until comfortably out of breath

Active recovery cool-down, see page 41
54 × several
60 until comfortably out of breath

Active recovery cool-down, see page 41
37 × 6
61 until muscles begin to tire
24 × 1
62 × 3
28, trying to bring head and shoulders off floor until muscles begin to tire
52 × several
63 × 4 each side
64 × several
65 × several
66 × up to 6 each leg
44 × several
67 × up to 5
68 × 1
58

59 **CALVES** *Start on all-fours, with legs fully extended and heels on ground. Now flex one knee and take weight onto other leg, pressing heel down into floor. Can you feel the stretch? Alternate from leg to leg in a nice steady rhythm 16 times.*

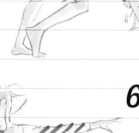

Excellent warm up for running as it stretches whole of back of leg

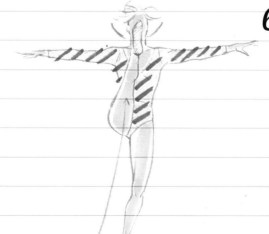

60 **KICKS** *Start jumping up and down lightly on both feet for 4 counts. Now bend one leg slightly as you kick other out to front, then down, then to side, then down, then to front again, then down, then to side again (8 counts). Go back to jumping lightly with both feet together for 4 counts and repeat with other leg. Continue until comfortably out of breath.*

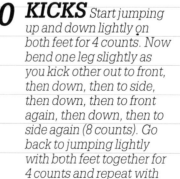

Aerobic exercises are strengtheners because they work the heart which is a muscle too and needs exercise just like any other muscle in the body . . .

61 UPPER BODY

A progression on the wall press-ups... Using a table makes exercise stronger because you lift more of body up against gravity. Do 4 press-ups, keeping back long and straight. Rest a moment, and repeat. How do you feel? Stop now if muscles feel well used; continue if you feel you can take more and stop when muscles begin to tire*.

*Note down how many sets of 4 you can do comfortably, without straining or dipping in back, for reference later...

ake sure able is firm and will not slip

A folded blanket beneath the heels gives them something to press against — makes for more of a stretch

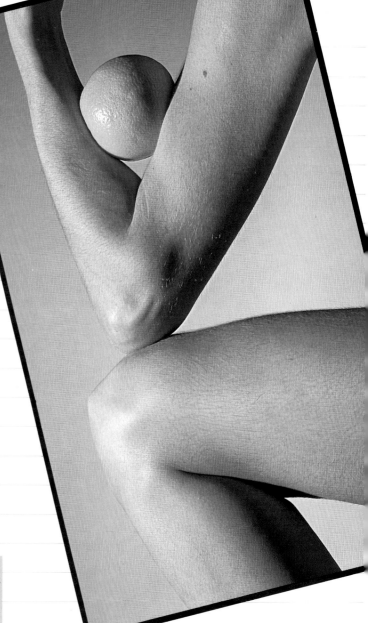

Muscle is composed of two types of fibre: the 'slow twitch' fibres are more suited to sustained strength, while the 'fast twitch' fibres are more suited to the strong, powerful movements that make for agility and speed. Both types of strength are important, which is why an exercise programme should alternate slow movements with quicker bursts of activity.

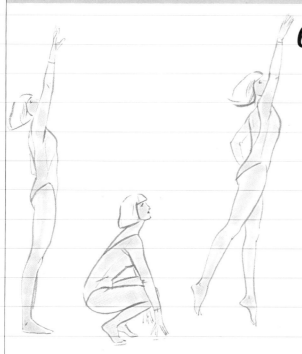

62 SQUAT JUMP

Stand by a wall, reach up with one hand and mark where you touch. Now crouch down and spring up to touch as high as possible above. Ask a friend to mark the spot. Try it 3 times, then take the best and measure distance between it and original mark.

The ability to push body weight up against gravity in one burst of energy is determined by fast-twitch muscle fibre.

Although height and weight should be taken into account for strictest accuracy, a measurement over 40 cm (16 ins) indicates you are likely to have a higher proportion of fast-twitch fibre...

The ratio of slow to fast-twitch muscle fibre does not change though it varies from individual to individual, determining which types of sport people are most suited. More slow-twitch fibres makes the endurance athlete, such as the marathon runner, while more fast-twitch fibres makes the more powerful shorter-distance athlete, such as the sprinter or the hurdler.

Find out which you are closest to with the squat jump test (exercise 62).

63 ABDOMEN

Lie on back with legs bent and feet flat on floor, arms about 30 cm (12 ins) away from body at sides. Breathe in. As you breathe out, take one hand across body to meet the other. Return to starting position and repeat to other side. Practise 4 times.

Excellent for tightening tummy

For extra strength, try making a noise as you breathe out. Some exercise physiologists maintain that this makes you 5 to 10 per cent stronger than staying silent...

Most of these strengtheners work on the front of the torso and not on the back because back muscles are almost invariably too tight and abdominal muscles too loose – penalties of poor posture and sedentary living. Concentrating on strengthening the front will tighten the tummy and help you gain greater length in the back, so improving your posture.

64 INNER THIGHS

Lie as before, with large cushion or pillow between knees. Breathe in. As you breathe out, do a pelvic tilt and press knees firmly together. Breathe in and release. Breathe out and repeat. Continue several times and finish by holding pelvic tilt, breathing normally and squeezing legs together several times quickly.

'The more feeble the body is, the more it commands; the stronger it is, the more it obeys...' Jean-Jacques Rousseau

65 OUTER THIGHS

Lie on side with legs stretched out, making sure body and legs are perfectly in line. Raise leg, keeping foot flexed and knee facing forwards. Do not aim for great height as this will mean turning leg out from hips and will defeat object of exercise. Lower leg half-way down and raise again. Continue until muscles begin to tire. Then lower leg and lift both legs off floor with feet together*. Take them as high as you can (at first this might only be an inch or two) and release. Turn over and repeat whole exercise with other leg.

BONUS
Tightens side of abdomen as well as outer thigh

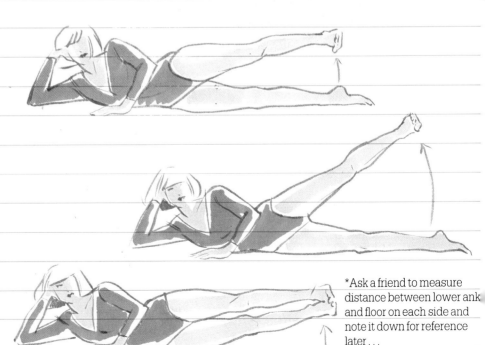

*Ask a friend to measure distance between lower ank and floor on each side and note it down for reference later...

66 BACKS OF THIGHS AND BUTTOCKS
Lie on front with pelvis supported by a cushion and forehead resting on hands in front of you. Take legs hip-width apart and bend them. Slowly lift them alternately up to 6 times each.

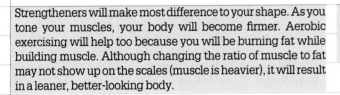

Strengtheners will make most difference to your shape. As you tone your muscles, your body will become firmer. Aerobic exercising will help too because you will be burning fat while building muscle. Although changing the ratio of muscle to fat may not show up on the scales (muscle is heavier), it will result in a leaner, better-looking body.

The most effective strengtheners ask muscles to shorten against gravity because they then have to work hard to support the weight of the body. Good examples: curl-ups, press-ups and this week's new front of thighs exercise (67).

67 FRONT OF THIGHS
Kneel with legs hip-width apart and arms out straight in front at shoulder level. Breathe in. As you breathe out, do a pelvic tilt and lean back until you can feel thighs working strongly to maintain position. Breathe in and come up. Practise up to 8 times

Muscles become sore and stiff through a build-up of metabolites – by-products of muscle contraction. These are carried away from the muscle by tiny blood capillaries. If a muscle is contracted for a long time, the capillaries are constricted, the blood cannot move freely and metabolites build up. After a while, the muscle will not be able to contract properly and the whole body may feel weak and stiff. Help prevent this by holding each position no longer than is comfortable and by warming down well after exercise…

Excellent strengthener as entire weight of body is supported by muscles working at front of thigh.

68 THIGHS
Still kneeling, bring knees together and take feet apart. Sit down between feet, if you can, and place one hand under each foot. Do a pelvic tilt and go back onto elbows, one at a time. Slowly lower head back. If you feel you can go further, slide arms out sideways and lower body onto floor, still maintaining pelvic tilt. You should feel no pain or squeezing in your lower back as you do this. Eventually this position becomes very relaxing.

If it's painful to sit between feet, sit on a cushion and let stretch come in that position; don't continue any further and relax as last week.

WEEK 8: AEROBICS

It is the mixture that makes exercise effective – activity with stillness, strength with suppleness, effort with easy movement . . .

Aerobics, a craze which has already collected more than its fair share of casualties, can defeat rather than enhance total fitness if carried out to the exclusion of everything else. As a part (an important part) but not the all, aerobics is great for working heart and lungs and enjoyable with it, provided that you build up gradually, as here.

All aerobic movements learned so far are now combined to make one continuous 4-minute sequence. Extending overall aerobic exercising time is important because it is the steady, sustained type of activity that produces the best benefits for heart and health.

This week's programme

Preliminaries
32 × several
69 × several
53 × several
34 × 8 each side
59 × 16
70
71
**Active recovery
   cool-down,** see page 41
37 × 6
61 until muscles begin to tire
28 until muscles begin to tire
52 × several
63 × several
64 × several
65 × several
66 × up to 6 each leg
44 × several
39, or with one leg bent
   38, × 1
30 × several
58

Aerobics literally means 'with air'. If you cannot sustain an activity for more than a minute or so – sprinting, swimming flat out and running upstairs are all good examples – the exercise is anaerobic because the demand outstrips the supply and builds up an 'oxygen debt' which leaves you breathless and gasping for air.

While aerobic exercise is steadier than anaerobic exercise and can be sustained comfortably for a reasonable time, it must also be vigorous enough to raise heart beat sufficiently to give a training effect. To begin with very gentle levels of activity, such as brisk walking, may do this but, as you get fitter, you will need to step up the pace.

69 **SIDES** *Stand with legs wide apart. Make sure pelvis is centered. Now take weight over onto one side straightening other knee and reaching up with arm as you go. Repeat several times from side to side in a good steady rhythm until the thighs begin to tire.*

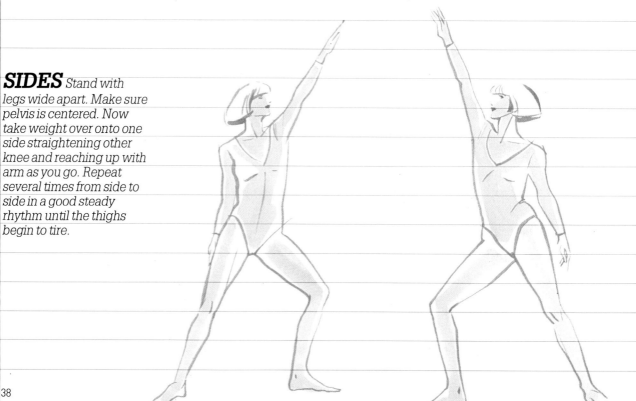

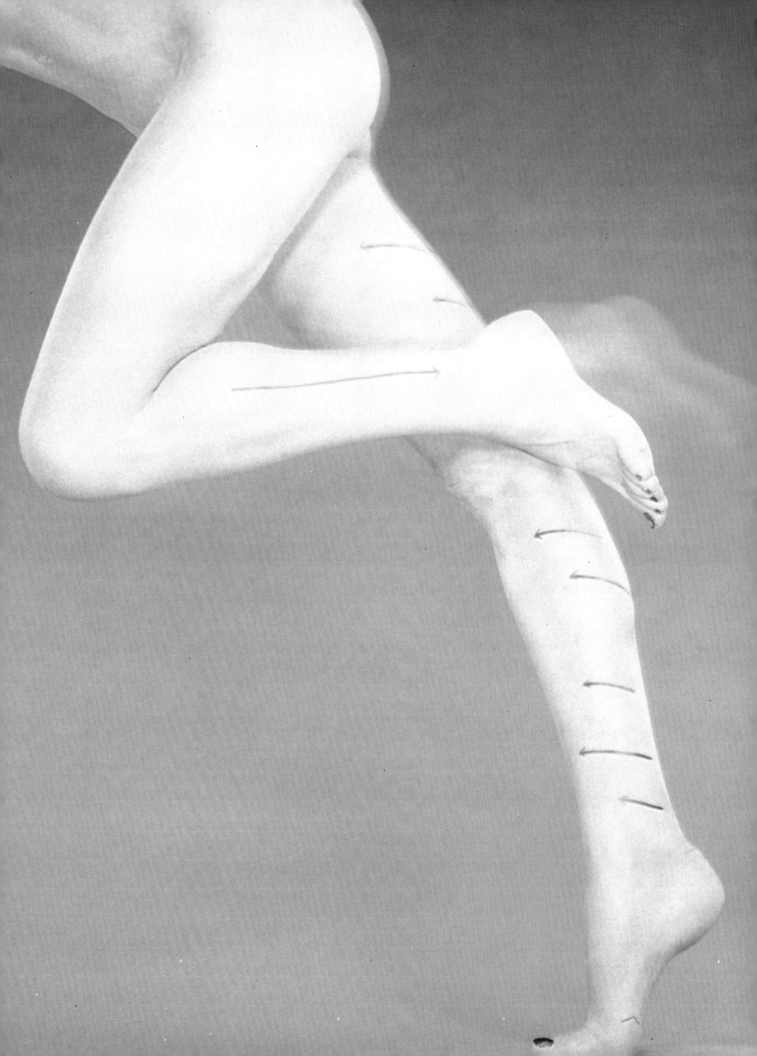

70 PULSE *Set aside one day each week and take pulse 3 times: before you start exercising, at the height of activity (just before you start cooling down) and again 10 minutes later.*

To take your pulse: locate it on the thumb side at the base of your left wrist. Curl your fingers – not your thumb – on the pulse and, using a stop watch or second hand on an ordinary watch, count *for 20 seconds. Multiply by 3 for a minute's count.*

Determine your maximum heart rate by taking your age from 220 (heart beats per minute). Aim to increase your fitness by sending your pulse rate up to between 70 and 85 per cent of maximum.

Gauge how much exercise is right for you by taking your pulse

If you take longer than 10 minutes to reduce pulse to normal, you have exercised too hard . . .

When you exercise aerobically, the lungs take in more air and the heart beats faster to send more oxygenated blood to the muscles for energy. With regular aerobic exercise, the heart actually becomes more efficient and sends more blood with each beat, so it does not need to beat as fast. This training effect can be monitored very easily by taking your pulse regularly, as indicated *left*.

See how much fitter you are getting by noticing a drop in your resting pulse rate (it may be as much as 10 beats or even more); by finding how much harder you have to work to get your exercise pulse up to target (your body's way of telling you your heart muscle is getting stronger and your cardiovascular endurance is improving); and by noticing how much closer your third reading (exercise 70) is to normal each time.

71 SEQUENCE *Start by running on the spot, padding from foot to foot and gradually getting higher (1 minute). Then reverse movement, so you are bringing feet back instead of forwards (30 seconds). Now combine them, running forwards for 8 steps and back for 8; repeat 4 times (1 minute). Regain your breath a bit* *with side lunges (30 seconds) and then go into side kicks (15 seconds), jump kicks with straight leg (15 seconds), star jumps (15 seconds) and twist jumps (15 seconds). If at any stage you feel out of breath, slow down and return to the quiet padding before you start building up the intensity again.*

Good quality training shoes are useful because they provide good support, help prevent jarring. They should be well cushioned with at least 1.5 cm (¾ in) under the heel and 1 cm (½ in) under the sole. Once feet and legs get stronger, you may find you don't need them – but you must have a good sprung surface if working barefoot.

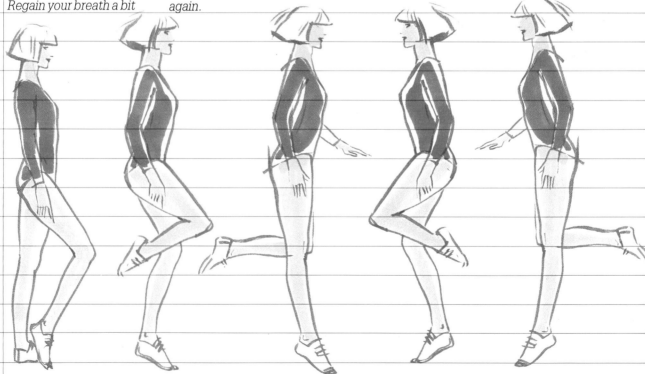

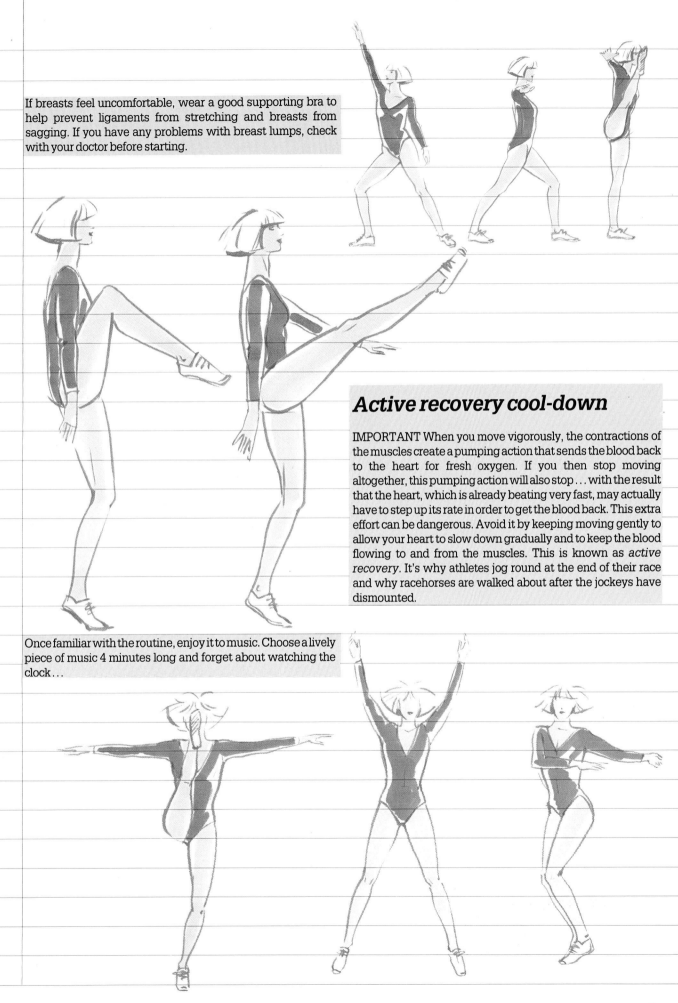

If breasts feel uncomfortable, wear a good supporting bra to help prevent ligaments from stretching and breasts from sagging. If you have any problems with breast lumps, check with your doctor before starting.

Active recovery cool-down

IMPORTANT When you move vigorously, the contractions of the muscles create a pumping action that sends the blood back to the heart for fresh oxygen. If you then stop moving altogether, this pumping action will also stop . . . with the result that the heart, which is already beating very fast, may actually have to step up its rate in order to get the blood back. This extra effort can be dangerous. Avoid it by keeping moving gently to allow your heart to slow down gradually and to keep the blood flowing to and from the muscles. This is known as *active recovery*. It's why athletes jog round at the end of their race and why racehorses are walked about after the jockeys have dismounted.

Once familiar with the routine, enjoy it to music. Choose a lively piece of music 4 minutes long and forget about watching the clock . . .

WEEK 9: WEIGHTS

Working with weights demands more from muscles, multiplies benefits, accelerates results … but make sure you can work with your own body weight first. Try these exercises on their own and add weights only if and when they become comfortable.

All strengthening exercises work on an *overloading* principle; to exercise a muscle effectively you must overload it by working it harder than usual. While straightforward strengtheners are fine to begin with, benefits decrease once muscles become stronger. So overload again, this time with weights.

This week's programme

Preliminaries
32 × several
69 × several
53 × several
34, bouncing a little further for 3 counts to each side, × 4 each side
72 × 6 rotations
59 × 16
71

Active recovery cool-down, see page 41
37, gently bouncing 3 times as you lower × 4
28, with arms folded in front until muscles begin to tire
52 × several
63, lifting shoulders off floor until muscles begin to tire
73 × 6 at each level
74 × 8 each leg
65, adding weights until muscles begin to tire
75 × up to 8
66, with weights and legs straight up to 8 each leg
16, leaving weights on for more swing × several
39, or with one leg bent **38**, × 1
30 × several
58

72 SHOULDERS
Strap a 0.5 kg (1 lb) weight to each wrist or improvise with food cans of an equivalent weight held in the hand. Stand with arms outstretched at chin level and rotate arms backwards 6 times.

Strap-on weights attach to wrists and ankles and can be bought from any sports shop and many department stores. Or improvise with food cans held in the hand and an old sock filled with sand tied loosely around the ankle. Start with weights of 0.5 kg (1 lb) each and work up to 1.5 kg (3 lb). That's your maximum: after that add repetitions, not weight …

73 CHEST
Lie on back with knees bent and weights strapped to wrists or held in the hand. Extend arms sideways at shoulder level. Breathe in. Breathe out as you bring weights up and cross arms over in front. Breathe in as you lower them. Practise 6 times and then repeat whole exercise at eye and waist levels in order to work every part of pectoral muscles.

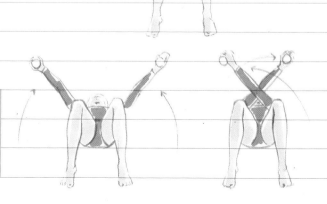

Weights can be used to build muscle strength or endurance. *Strength*, achieved by using heavy weights and few repetitions, strengthens muscle in a few specific areas and builds bulk – the type of training weightlifters do. *Endurance*, achieved by using light weights and many repetitions, tones and tightens the entire muscle and does not add bulk.

Attaching weights to wrists and ankles increases the toning effect of the exercise because greater resistance must be overcome as the arm or leg is lifted against gravity.

74 FRONT OF THIGHS

Sit on a table so that thighs are well supported up to knee, with a 0.5 kg (1 lb) weight strapped round each ankle. Breathe in. As you breathe out, slowly lift one leg up until it is completely straight. Breathe in and lower. Practise, alternating legs, 16 times.

Can be excellent for strengthening knees, particularly if weak, but consult your doctor first if you do have a problem.

If you can't extend leg fully, try exercise without weights.

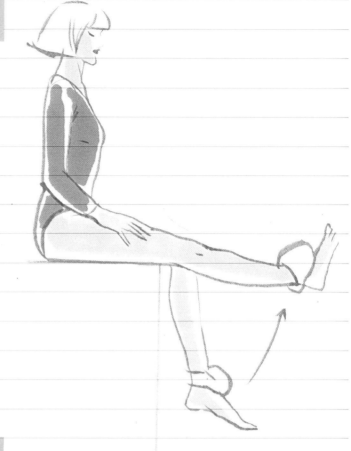

Curl-ups are one of the best tummy tighteners because the muscles have to contract from a position of maximum length as you bring your body up against gravity. Doing them this week with your arms folded in front will make the exercise stronger, as you cannot use arms to help pull you up.

75 INNER THIGHS

Lie on back with arms outstretched and a 0.5 kg (1 lb) weight attached to each ankle. Slip hands beneath pelvis to ensure that lower back remains pressed into floor. Raise legs by bending them first into chest and then straightening them up. Take them slowly apart as wide as you can and then bring them together again equally slowly. Practise up to 6 times.

If back hurts, work at Feldenkrais mobility sequence for spine, page 122, and skip this for the moment.

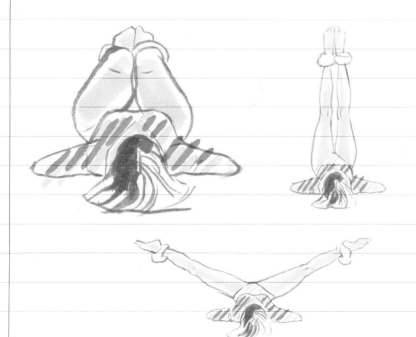

WEEK 10: BALANCE

Balance, the keynote of an effective exercise programme, is also an important aspect of fitness in its own right. Do you know how good yours is?

Don't be disheartened if, having completed the tests, the answer is not very good. No-one need be stuck with a poor sense of balance. It can be improved by more attention to posture, and by relaxation techniques or meditation to help calm the mind. Practice can be helpful too. But don't confuse practice with effort. Effort, can interfere with balance by overriding subliminal messages coming from the brain and central nervous system. Stop trying so hard and you may do better.

This week's programme

Preliminaries
57 × 3 mins each foot
56 × 1
76 × several
77 × 1 each leg
69 × several
53 × several
72 × 6 rotations
24 × 1
78 × 3
59 × 16
79
Active recovery cool-down, see page 41
37 × 4
28 until muscles begin to tire
52 × several
63 until muscles begin to tire
80 × several at each stage
73 × 6 at each level
65 × several
75 × several
39, or with one leg bent
    38, × 1
58
77 × 1 each leg

76 **BALANCE** *Stand with feet hip-width apart and shift weight from foot to foot to help you assess which side of your body is carrying most weight. Now imagine you are on a tightrope. Stand well with spine lengthened and both feet together. Lift one heel. Imagine someone is pulling that knee forwards with an invisible piece of string. Then take that foot and place it in front of the other. Transfer weight onto forward foot and immediately lift back foot and place that in front,* *again imagining someone is pulling knee forwards. Practise taking several steps along your tightrope. Note breathing and position of head. Now try walking backwards, maintaining length in back and not turning head round to see where you are going. Take several steps backwards, then stand with feet together again. Does balance feel different?*

Notice that when walking you maintain balance by having all your weight on one foot at a time.

How straight is your tightrope? Try exercise again with eyes shut. Mark where you start and take same number of steps forwards and backwards. Where do you finish?

As you need to be calm and unflustered to balance well, it can be a very good barometer of your state of mind. It is sure to be affected if overtired or agitated and is often less good before a period; increased clumsiness and liability to accidents are now recognized symptoms of pre-menstrual tension. So don't be surprised if it seems easier some days than others.

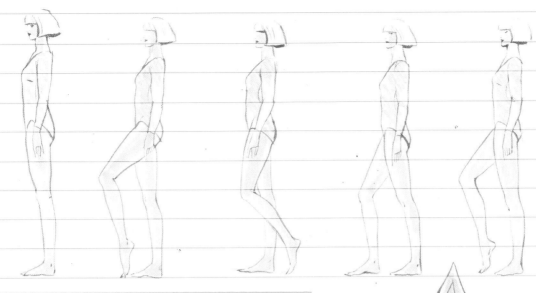

LOOK ON BALANCE AS AN ACTIVE, RATHER THAN PASSIVE, QUALITY... However still and balanced a body seems, it is never static. A dynamic distribution of energy in the nerves and muscle of the body will be taking place all the time to keep it upright, prevent it toppling over. The slightest shift in posture and thousands of tiny adjustments will be made...

77 | **BALANCE** *Stand on one leg and lift other foot onto inner thigh, using hands to help you. Place it as high as you can. Now lift arms to ceiling and remain in this position for as long as you can. Can you close eyes and still keep balance? Change sides and repeat.*

This 'tree pose' may be easier on one side than the other; if so, practise weaker side more often.

78 | **LEGS** *Stand well with feet together and arms by side. Bring arms up to shoulder level and then lift heels. Slowly go down into squat position. Can you go right the way down, so that bottom is resting on heels, and up again, without losing balance? You must go all the way up with heels lifted, only returning them to ground when completely upright. Try 3 times keeping smooth rhythm.*

CAUTION Don't go all the way down if knees are weak.

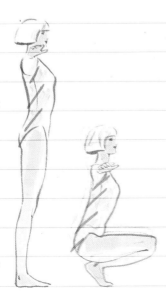

If you can remain in pose with eyes closed for 1 minute, your balance is good

45

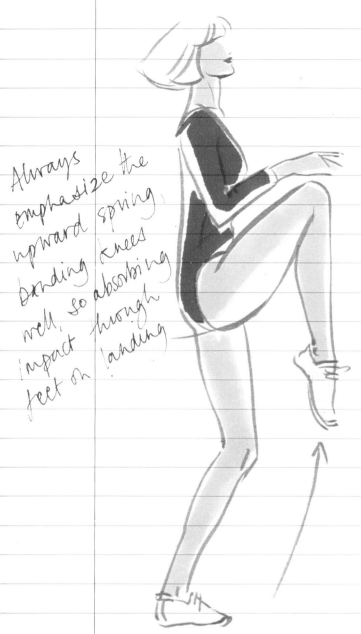

Always emphasize the upward spring, bending knees well, so absorbing impact through feet on landing

79 AEROBIC

Now try lifting knees really high as you spring from foot to foot when running on the spot. Ensure you are getting a good height by placing arms out in front, as shown, and bringing thighs up to touch. Resist temptation to bring hands down to meet them! Continue until comfortably out of breath and then wind down a little with some easy jogging and padding before continuing aerobic sequence. Extend more energetic parts of sequence by a few seconds to bring total up to 5 minutes.

REMEMBER Balance improves with physical confidence and physical confidence improves with fitness.

80 BALANCE

Sit with knees bent and feet flat. Rock from side to side and then round in a circle so that you can feel your two 'sitting' bones. When weight is evenly balanced on both, you will know pelvis is centered. Place hands under heels and lift both legs up, with knees still bent. When you feel stable, rock gently back and forth several times.

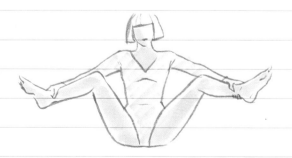

Then try this balancing trick. Breathe in and do a pelvic tilt. As you breathe out, lift arms and legs into air to make a wide V-shape. Can you maintain your balance in this position?

Practice and patience will help if you can't achieve this right away; take time on each stage so you learn to balance steadily before straightening legs.

Does balance improve after activity? Try the 'tree pose' before and after the programme and see. If balance improves, exercise is having exactly the right benefits for you, helping you to feel revitalized and calm at the same time. If balance does not improve, ask yourself whether you are rushing into the exercises – and, if so, take them more slowly.

WEEK 11: COORDINATION

Coordination, like balance, is an aspect of fitness we can all improve on. A lucky few may be blessed with exceptional coordination, but the rest of us have to learn to move our bodies well. From the infant guiding spoon to mouth to the tennis player returning a ball, the lesson is the same: coordination, like any other skill, is to be mastered with practice.

The key to doing these exercises well – and most sports too – lies as much in the mind as in the body. Keep a relaxed, non-judging attitude. Worrying about your performance will cause muscles to tense up and shorten, leading to awkward jerky movements which will interfere with your coordination and may even inhibit movement altogether. Let your body find its own rhythm and you will feel the movements becoming smoother and easier.

This week's programme
Preliminaries
77 × 1 each leg
56 × 1
42 × 1
81 × 1
69, changing rhythm every 4 lunges to bend opposite knee to outstretched arm × several
53 × several
72 × 6 rotations
24 × 1
61 until muscles begin to tire
82 × several
59 × 16
83
Active recovery cool-down, see page 41
84 × several
28 until muscles begin to tire
52 × several
85 until muscles begin to tire
86
87
65 × several
75 × up to 6
88 × 4
58

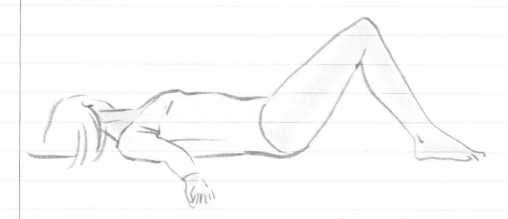

81 HEAD AND PELVIS

Lie on back with knees bent and feet flat on floor, as for pelvic clock. Visualize a clock on the back of your head with 12 o'clock at top, 6 o'clock where spine joins skull, 3 o'clock under left ear and 9 o'clock under right ear.
a. *Now read instructions for pelvis on page 27 and perform them with head.*

Take time, do them thoroughly and rest often.
b. *Do you notice that your pelvis moves in conjunction with your head? Move them both together from 6 to 12 and back again several times. Now move pelvis to 6 and head to 12; pelvis to 12 and head to 6. Repeat several times and rest.*

c. *Move pelvis and head to 12 and make a complete clockwise circle with both, travelling slowly and gently around clock. Rest. Travel in an anti-clockwise direction equally slowly. Rest.*
d. *Finally, for a gentle but challenging lesson in coordination, move pelvis and head to 12 and let pelvis travel in an*

anti-clockwise direction while head travels in a clockwise direction. Do this slowly and gently. Stop and rest when you get confused and then start again. Repeat several times and then reverse the direction. Rest. Stand up and walk around. How does your pelvis feel? Your head? Your neck? Your back?

82 COORDINATION

Stand with arms outstretched at shoulder level and lift foot about 5 cm (2 ins) off floor. Now rotate foot as you move it out towards back in an anti-clockwise direction. Bring it in again, this time rotating it in a clockwise direction. Try it several times with each foot. Then try bringing arms forwards, rotating hands in an anti-clockwise direction, and backwards, rotating hands smoothly in a clockwise direction. Practise several times. Then put both together. Repeat several times or until you get it right.

Stop trying, so hard!

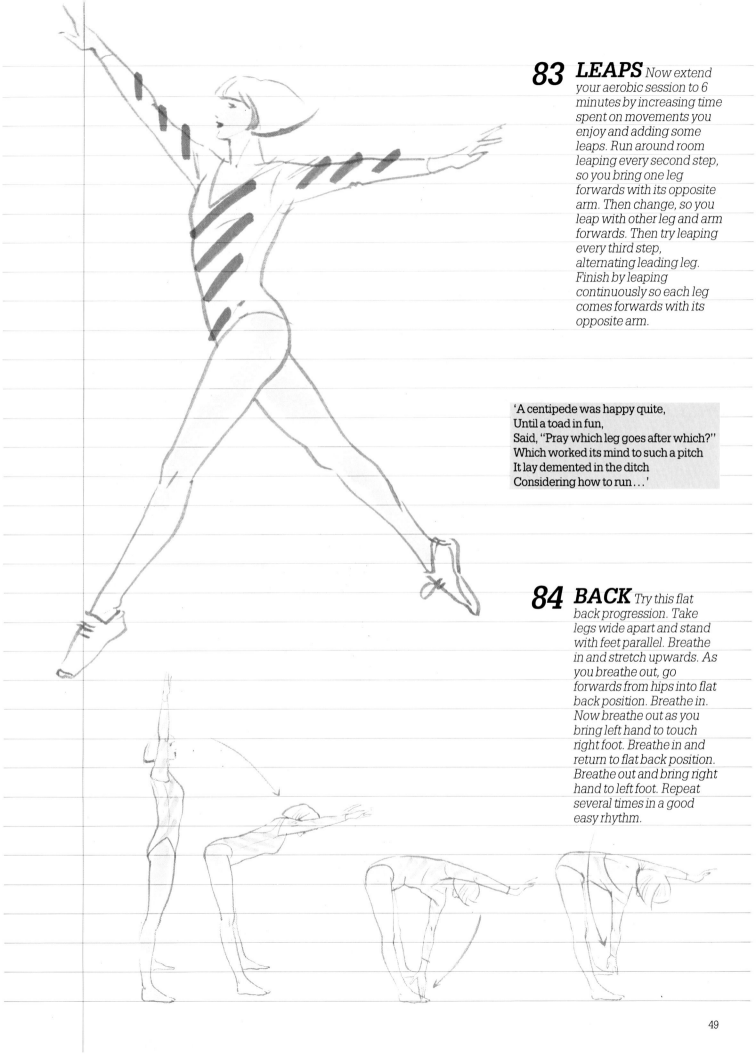

83 LEAPS *Now extend your aerobic session to 6 minutes by increasing time spent on movements you enjoy and adding some leaps. Run around room leaping every second step, so you bring one leg forwards with its opposite arm. Then change, so you leap with other leg and arm forwards. Then try leaping every third step, alternating leading leg. Finish by leaping continuously so each leg comes forwards with its opposite arm.*

'A centipede was happy quite,
Until a toad in fun,
Said, "Pray which leg goes after which?"
Which worked its mind to such a pitch
It lay demented in the ditch
Considering how to run...'

84 BACK *Try this flat back progression. Take legs wide apart and stand with feet parallel. Breathe in and stretch upwards. As you breathe out, go forwards from hips into flat back position. Breathe in. Now breathe out as you bring left hand to touch right foot. Breathe in and return to flat back position. Breathe out and bring right hand to left foot. Repeat several times in a good easy rhythm.*

49

85 ABDOMEN
Lie on back with legs bent and feet flat on floor. Clasp hands behind head. Breathe in. As you breathe out bring right knee towards left elbow, letting other leg come off floor as comfortable. Breathe in and release. Breathe out and bring left knee towards right elbow. Continue in a good rhythm until muscles feel well used.

Exercise becomes harder as you take straight leg lower

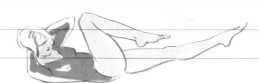

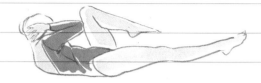

86 LEGS
Lie on back. Bend one knee so foot is flat on floor. Stretch other out and raise it about 10 cm (4 ins) off floor. Beat it vigorously in air for 16 counts. Repeat with other leg.

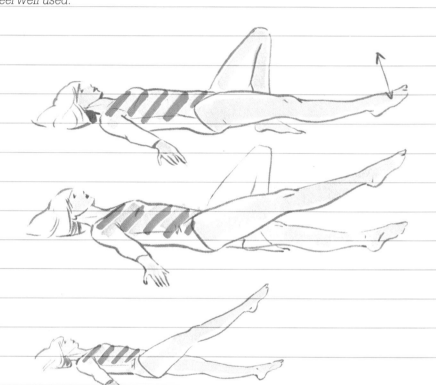

87 LEGS
Now try previous exercise again, but this time as you beat one leg bend and straighten other every 4 counts. Change legs and repeat.

88 BACK AND BUTTOCKS
Lie on front with pelvis resting on a cushion, and forehead resting on hands in front. Raise both legs bending knees and bring them out to sides, rotating feet inwards as you go. Return them to centre, rotating feet outwards. Repeat twice and then try rotating feet in opposite directions as you bring legs out and in again.

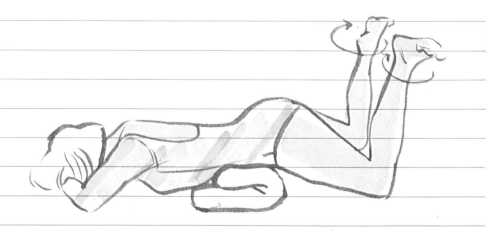

Because coordination is a function of brain as well as body, mental relaxation techniques can often help. If you find these exercises difficult, try them again after the relaxation and see if you improve . . .

WEEK 12: HALF-TERM EXAMS

Half-way through, and time to see how well you are doing. Although competition plays no part in getting fit, a sense of progress and achievement does. So run through these tests to see how much you have improved and to gain fresh incentive for the next 12 weeks.

Some benefits should be clear already. How do you feel compared to when you started? If the answer is stronger and fitter, more energetic and less tired, more in tune with your body and its needs – then you pass with honours because that is what exercising is all about.

These tests assess the specific aspects of fitness that add up to true health – posture, flexibility, strength, balance, stamina, the ability to relax... Excelling in just some of them is not enough, you must be up to scratch on every one before you can consider yourself in really good shape.

This week's programme

Preliminaries
32 × several
69 × several
53 × several
34 × 8 each side
89 × 1 each side
59 × 16
83, with pulse test (70, see note)

Active recovery
cool-down, see page 41
84 × several
90 × 1
91
92
52 × several
85 until muscles begin to tire
65, with progress test 93, × several
75 × up to 6
94 × 1
95 × 1
96 × 1
97 × 1
44 × several
58
98 × 1 min

Examine yourself on one day only this week and use the others to run through the basic programme, concentrating on weak areas...

89 SIDES *Put palm of hand against a wall at shoulder level and, standing sideways, try to stretch other hand over head to touch, without twisting at waist. Repeat to other side.*

You should find this easy; if not, practise until you do.

you should find this easy – if not practise until you do

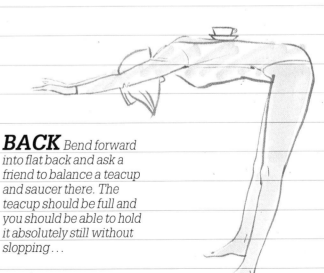

90 BACK *Bend forward into flat back and ask a friend to balance a teacup and saucer there. The teacup should be full and you should be able to hold it absolutely still without slopping...*

These exams differ from the academic type in 3 ways. First you are the only person taking part; second there is no examiner – you should *know* if you have made the grade; and, third, there are no prizes – simply greater confidence and well-being.

51

91 UPPER BODY

Do table press-ups in sets of 4, with a small rest in between, and continue until muscles begin to tire. How many sets of 4 can you do maintaining perfect technique – i.e. without straining or dipping in the back? Turn back to week 7 (exercise 61) and check your progress.

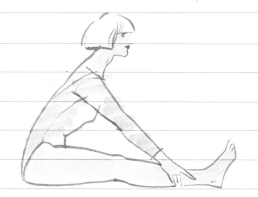

92 ABDOMEN

How many curl-ups can you do comfortably with arms folded in front? Turn back to week 2 (exercise 28) and check progress by seeing how well you did on the preliminary stage of this exercise. If you can do as many or more of this more demanding progression, you are doing very well.

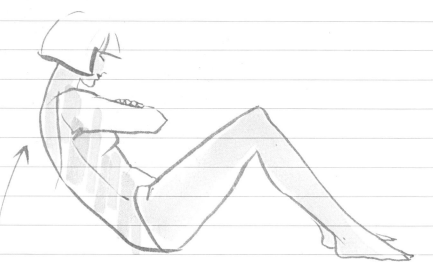

93 OUTER THIGHS

Lie on side, supported by elbow, and take both legs up in air as high as you can. When you feel quite stable, ask a friend to measure the distance between lower ankle and floor on both sides and then turn back to week 7 (exercise 65) and check your progress.

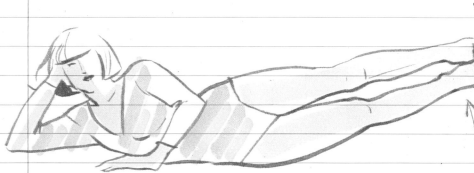

94 BALANCE

Can you now manage to do the V-trick with both legs fully extended? If not, practise until you can.

CAUTION Not for weak backs

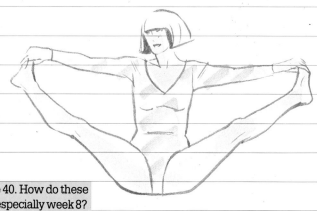

Take your pulse 3 times as directed on page 40. How do these readings differ from the previous 4 weeks – especially week 8? If both resting and post-exercise pulse have dropped by several beats, you are doing well . . .

95 **BACK** *Sit with bottom against a wall and soles of feet together as close to you as possible. Place hands on ankles and lengthen spine upwards as much as possible. Pull thighs downwards and ask a friend to measure distance between knees and floor. Now turn back to week 1 (exercise 14) and see how you have progressed. Come away from wall and repeat test with back unsupported and take another measurement. If this is less than your original, and your back is quite straight, you are doing very well indeed . . .*

If you can't get knees below waist level, practise hip loosening exercises in Therapeutics section, page 123, until you can.

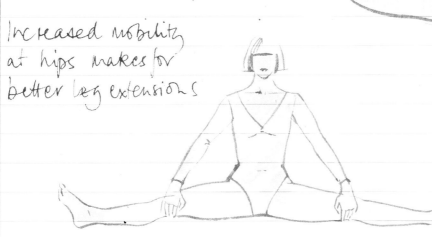

Increased mobility at hips makes for better leg extensions

96 **BACK** *Sitting on floor, take legs apart until you feel a good stretch in inner thighs. Lengthen back well and, if you cannot maintain position with spine lengthened, bring legs in until you can. Ask a friend to measure distance between feet and then turn back to week 1 (exercise 15) to check your progress.*

Exercises 95, 96, 97 test for mobility in the hips as much as for strength, and length, in the back: lengthening the spine allows the hip joint to rotate outwards more easily (95), giving better leg extensions (96) and enabling the back to bend further from the hips (97).

97 **BACK** *Turn back to week 3 (exercise 39) and look at the dotted line you made on the diagram. Now sit sideways on to a mirror with feet out in front as before. Lengthen well up spine as you breathe in and, as you breathe out, bend forwards from hips keeping back quite straight. Can you go further than before?*

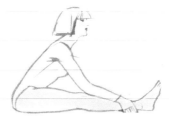

98 **BALANCE** *Has your balance improved over the last 2 weeks? Try the 'tree pose' (exercise 77) with eyes closed and ask a friend to time you. If you can maintain position without wobbling or opening eyes for a full minute you are doing very well.*

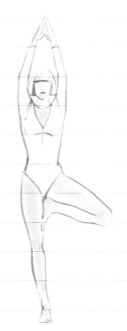

WEEK 13: SHAPERS I

If you know what your weak points are, and why you have them, you are already half-way towards a more evenly proportioned body. The next two weeks' exercises can take you the other half of the way by showing how you can help overcome them.

The length and basic shape of the legs, the width of the shoulders, waist and hips and the size of the breasts are all genetically determined. Although these basic proportions cannot be changed, you can do a tremendous amount to make your body the firmest and best-looking possible of its type.

It is not just any old exercise that firms and tightens, *it is the right type*. Flab, the bit that dieting leaves behind, can spoil the line of the slimmest body. Because it collects in areas of the body that are not frequently used, such as the underside of the upper arm and innerside of the thigh, you will need some well-chosen exercises *in addition* to a balanced diet and an active lifestyle in order to keep in shape. Now to work...

This week's programme
Preliminaries
32 × several
69 × several
53 × several
34 × 8 each side
99 × several
100 × 8
59 × 16
83
Active recovery
 cool-down, see page 41
84 × several
101 × up to 8
102 × 4
51 × 1 each side
103 × 4
52 × several
85 until muscles begin to tire
73 × 6 at each level
64 × several
66 × up to 8 each leg
39 × 1
68 × 1

Place thumbs just below base of skull to feel neck muscles tighten

99 | **CHIN** *Clasp hands at back of head, as shown, and press head back while pulling forwards with hands at same time. Repeat several times.*

This week, start with some healthy self-appraisal. Areas that can be improved upon will determine where you need to get to work. Do the relevant exercises 3 to 5 times a week throughout the rest of the programme, and you will soon see an improvement. Expect to notice real differences after 12 weeks...

Think back to front for double chins: jawline is kept trim by muscles at the back, not the front, of the neck.

100 UPPER ARMS

Stand in flat back position, with feet hip-width apart and knees bent. Bend arms forwards so that upper arms are parallel to floor and elbow is at a right angle. Breathe in. As you breathe out, straighten arms backwards fully extending elbows. Breathe in and return to starting position. Practise 8 times, keeping movement controlled – don't just fling arms back.

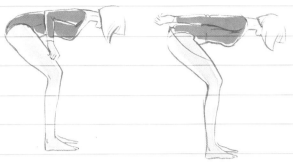

When exercise is comfortable use weights and gradually build repetitions.

The biceps, continually brought into action by any movement that brings hands towards shoulders, such as lifting, are always firm; but the triceps which lie on the underside of the upper arm are often a problem, being brought into action only when the arm extends backwards. This movement can become an effective tightening exercise when weights are used (100). Other helpful exercises: 73 and 91.

101 UPPER BODY

Kneel on all-fours and walk hands forwards until your back makes a nice straight line all the way from back of knees to back of head. Breathe in. As you breathe out, bend elbows and lower body to floor, keeping back straight. (It is useful to do this sideways on to a mirror to begin with to check back is flat and not sagging in middle.) Breathe in and raise up again. Practise up to 8 times in a good steady rhythm.

Firms arms, chest and upper back – areas most women don't exercise enough.

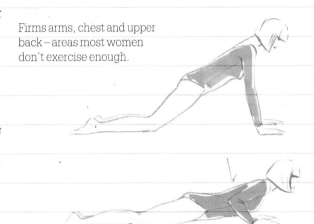

Do not rest body on floor between press-ups

Chest exercises won't increase breast size or firm up breasts that have already sagged because the breast is not a muscle; but they can do much to keep breasts firm and lifted by working the underlying supporting muscles. Helpful exercises: 7, 73, 101, 102.

102 SIDES

This excellent exercise works the latissimus dorsi muscles at side and helps counteract flabbiness around bra strap area – a very common problem. You will need a strong partner and a broom handle. Kneel on floor and hold broom handle with hands well apart and arms fully extended above head. Ask partner to stand behind you with his hands on centre of handle. Breathe in. As you breathe out, gradually pull handle down as he resists. The whole movement should take about 10 seconds and handle should be pulled down until it touches back of neck. Practise 4 times.

Experiment a little to establish how much resistance partner should apply

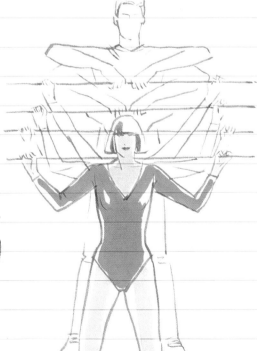

103 **ABDOMEN** Lie on back with legs bent and arms at sides. Breathe in. As you breathe out, lift head off floor, pulling forwards with hands. Breathe in and return to floor. Breathe out and lift head and shoulders off floor. Breathe in and return. Breathe out and lift head, shoulders and ribcage off floor. Breathe in and return. Breathe out and come all the way up to a sitting position. Now curl all the way down to floor again, in stages as before, breathing out as you curl down, in as you come up ... Practise 4 times, remembering your breathing.

Thick waists are slimmed by bending and twisting movements. Helpful exercises: 34 and 51. Do several each time you exercise.

Weight training machines, such as those used by the Nautilus system*, can be great for conditioning under-used areas because they isolate specific muscle groups. If there is a Nautilus gym in your area, twice-weekly workouts would make an excellent supplement to these exercises.
*Now widely available in gyms in the UK and US.

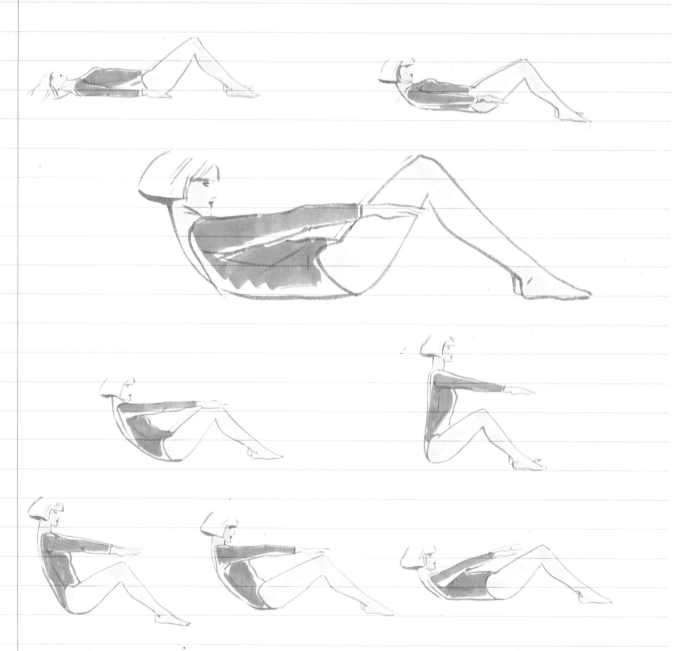

Work towards doing
this with arms
folded in front

The abdomen is wrapped in muscles which run vertically, horizontally and diagonally like the lines on the Union Jack. These soon become slack and weak through lack of use. Make the most of this natural built-in girdle by working each set of muscles (exercises 103, 65 and 85 respectively).

WEEK 14: SHAPERS II

The shaping-up theme continues. Attention, this week, on buttocks, hips and thighs. Remember to incorporate the relevant shapers from last week too . . .

104 | **BUTTOCKS AND HIPS** *Attach a light 0.5 kg (1 lb) weight to each ankle. Holding onto back of chair for support, transfer weight onto inside leg; now take leg out to side as far as possible, keeping foot flexed. Return to floor and rotate foot* outwards to angle of about 45° and then extend leg backwards in a straight line as far as comfortable, keeping back vertical and not arching or leaning forwards. Return leg to starting position. Practise 12 times, then change legs and repeat.

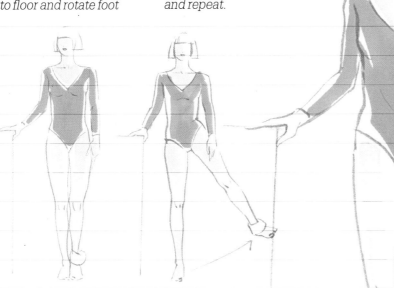

Firms slack buttock muscles at side, reduces bulge at hips

Back view . . . If buttocks hang over at the back or creep round to the sides, contributing to a bulge at the hips, they need firming. <u>Helpful exercises:</u> 104, if you cannot see a definite dent at the sides beneath the hips; 66 and 105 if your shape at the back is not firm and well defined.

105 | **BUTTOCKS** *Lie on back with legs falling gently outwards. Do a pelvic tilt and squeeze buttocks together several times. Then repeat, but this time hold each contraction for 6 counts before releasing. Practise several times.*

Buttock muscles soon respond to exercise

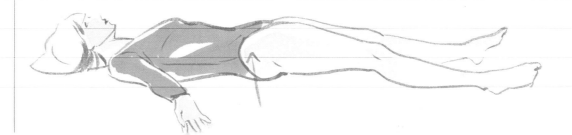

106 INNER THIGHS

Lie on back with knees bent, feet flat on floor. Place a football-sized ball between knees and squeeze quickly together 8 times. Then try 8 slower contractions, continuing to squeeze for 6 counts. Now place a smaller tennis-sized ball between knees and repeat exercise.

Using different sized balls works entire range of muscles

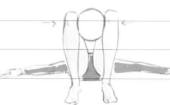
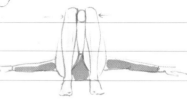

107 INNER THIGHS

Lie on side, as shown, with body in a straight line and knees facing forwards. Place upper foot on chair seat and point toes. Now flex lower foot and bring it up to meet the other. Hold for 3 counts and release. Practise 8 times, then turn over and change legs.

When comfortable add weight to lower ankle

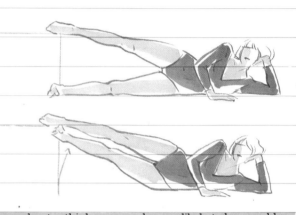

Inner and outer thighs are much more likely to be a problem than front or back because they are used for lateral movements and rotation only. The muscles at the front of thigh, which are used for forward motion, usually remain firm and toned even in the overweight. Helpful exercises for inner thighs: 64, 75, 106, 107...alternate for variety. Helpful exercises for outer thighs ('saddlebags'): 65 and 108.

108 OUTER THIGHS

Lie on side, supported by one elbow, with lower leg bent back at knee. Flex foot of upper leg and raise until it is parallel to floor. Hold for 6 slow counts and slowly lower. Repeat until muscles begin to tire, and then turn over and repeat with other leg.

When exercise is comfortable add weights to ankle

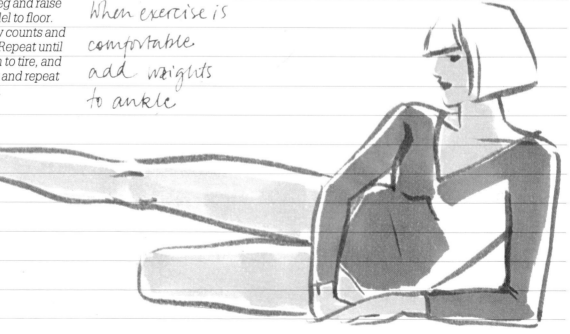

WEEK 15: MOBILITY

The freedom to move easily is one of our most basic freedoms and, very often, the one we think least about. But we should treasure it. Keeping mobile by being mobile can prevent any amount of stiffness later on.

Keeping mobile means taking each joint through its full range of movement every day (knees are the exception, see over), *not* contorting your body into strange shapes. It doesn't matter a bit whether you can do the splits or get your foot around your neck. These are gimmicks. But it does matter tremendously if you cannot move as and how you wish. There is nothing more demoralizing than a stiff, awkward body that protests every time you ask it to move.

As you work through the exercises this week, sense yourself becoming more supple. Results should be rewardingly swift. As your range of movement develops you may find yourself capable of more in other directions too: freedom from physical stiffness can lead to greater mental and emotional freedom...

This week's programme
Preliminaries
32 × several
69 × several
53 × several
24 × 3
109 × several
110 × 8 each direction
111 × 8 each leg
46 × 8 each leg
83
Active recovery
 cool-down, see page 41
74 × 4 each leg
103 × 4
52 × several
85 until muscles begin to tire
112
Active recovery
 cool-down, see page 41
113 until ankles and calves begin to tire
42 × 1
43, 44, 45 × several
114 × 3 each way
68 × 1
N.B. Remember to include Shapers from last two weeks where appropriate...

109 **ELBOWS** *Stand with feet about hip-width apart and a book, or flat object, in the palm of each hand. Now bring hands in towards you as you bend elbows out and stretch arms out again. Repeat smoothly several times.*

Don't clutch onto books – they should simply balance on the flat of your hand.

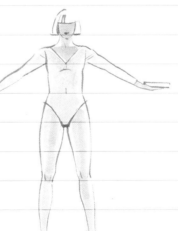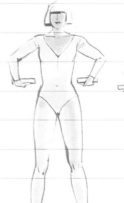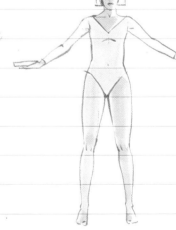

Thumbs should face back in both positions

You should do mobility work before aerobics and the stronger stretches and strengtheners because it helps you both to work more effectively and to guard against injury – particularly important in cold climates where joints tend to be stiff and need to be warmed up well before attempting anything more demanding.

110 SHOULDERS

Stand with feet about 60 cm (2 ft) apart. Hold a broom handle in front of you and lift it up to shoulder level. Raise one arm up above head, letting the other drop to waist. Now use both arms to take stick backwards as far as it will go. Then bring it down behind you so that shoulder blades are squeezed together. Continue round back to the front again, raising opposite arm to the one before. Practise 8 times in each direction. This exercise is much used by javelin throwers.

BONUS Improves coordination. As you get better change direction every 4 times, then every 2 . . .

Bring hands in as shoulders become more supple

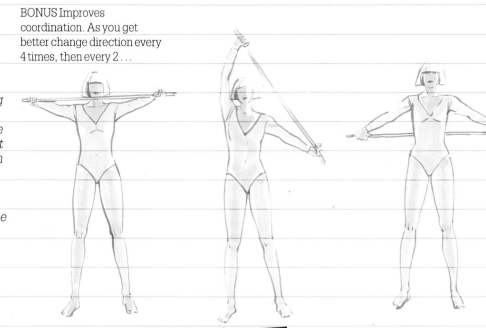

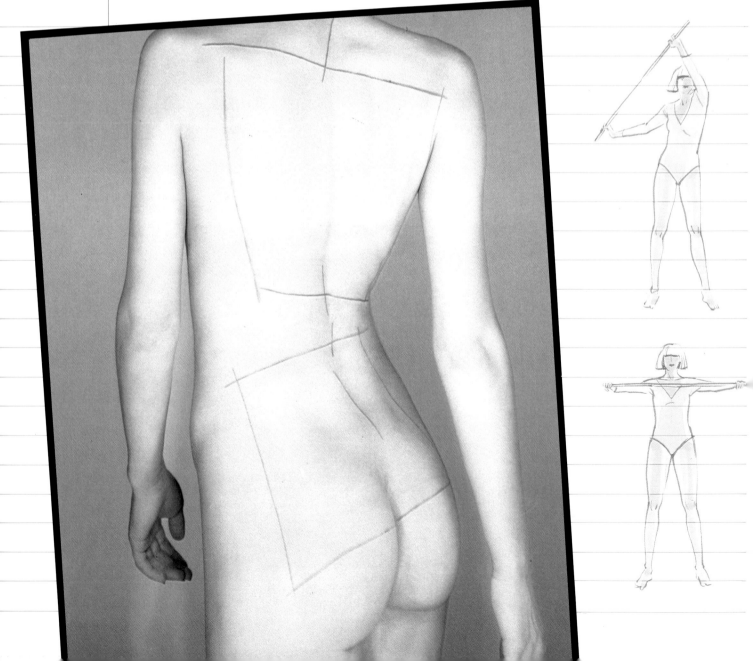

111 **HIPS** *Stand holding onto back of chair for support. Bend outside leg so thigh is parallel to floor and toes are pointed. Now make a wide circle with leg, keeping back vertical and feeling stretch on inside of hip as you bring leg right round to back. Return to starting position. Practise 8 times with each leg.*

Sense hip moving deep within socket as you bring leg backwards and forwards.

The straighter your back, the more hips must work.

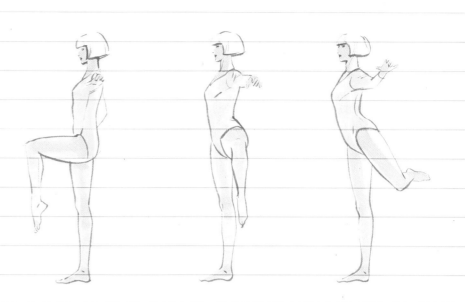

112 **AEROBIC SEQUENCE** *Add another, improvised, aerobic sequence to your routine. Pick a lively piece of music 4 minutes long, start and finish with gentle padding (see note) and then choose from aerobic movements you have already learned, adding new ones given here.*

a. Progress the twist jump so you are jumping with about one walking step between feet.

b. Try some scissor jumps, first straight forwards and then to diagonal, back to centre and then to other diagonal. Feet should be one walking pace apart.
c. Stand well with heels about 10cm (4ins) apart and spring up, landing with alternate feet forwards. Make sure that knees bend directly over toes and don't lean forwards: tuck pelvis under and jump up and down looking straight ahead.

What intensity of aerobic exercise is right for you? As you get fitter make it more demanding. Move faster and jump higher, always emphasizing the upward spring. If you begin to tire, slow down and go back to some gentle padding before increasing the pace again.

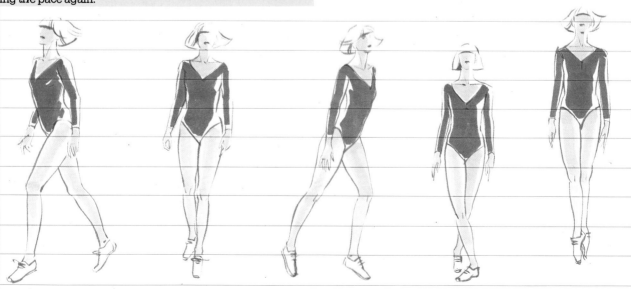

You will find that no mobility exercises are given for the knee because the knee is designed to work safely on one plane only (see page 123). This vulnerable joint is kept stable by the muscles at the front of the thigh. Strengthen these and you will help keep the knee trouble-free. Most effective strengthener: exercise 74. Try it this week holding the fully extended position for 4 counts before slowly lowering.

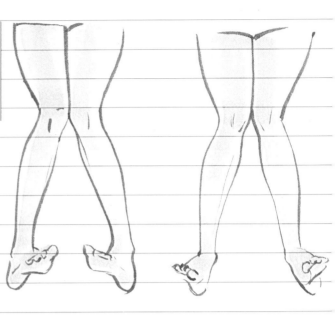

113 ANKLES

Sit on a chair with knees together and heels apart. Bring big toes together, trying to lift them up as much as possible. Then brush outwards along floor, pulling little toes up and pressing big toes down. Repeat until ankles and calves begin to tire.

TEST Can you raise big toes at least 15 cm (5 ins) when heels are on floor? If not, practise until you can. You will be able to lift toes higher as ankles become more mobile.

Weak feet and ankles are easily injured. Strong, springy ones make you feel agile and lively and improve your balance. Exercises that increase mobility at ankles will help strengthen them and improve posture too ...

114 SPINE

Sit with legs crossed and take right leg back, so that left foot is by right knee. You should be well balanced and able to feel both 'sitting' bones beneath you. Stretch left hand behind you, resting on fingers. Raise right arm and twist to left, bending from hips. Try to keep hips level and facing front as you reach forwards to diagonal and sweep round to right, changing position of arms as you go through centre. If you can, drop back onto elbow and look behind you. Then sweep back again, going forwards as far as possible and round to opposite side. Practise 3 times, then reverse legs and repeat.

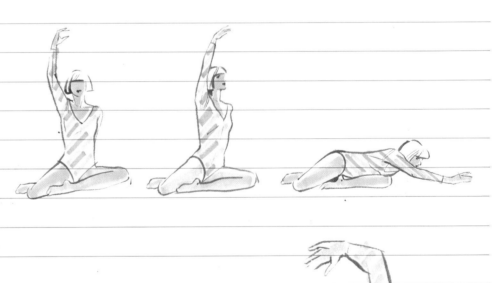

This is borrowed from contemporary dance, and stabilizes hips to give good twist in spine.

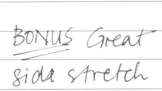

BONUS Great side stretch

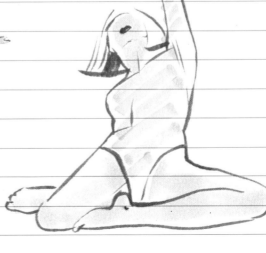

62

WEEK 16: DŌ-IN

The new-wave holistic approach to medicine underlines the interaction of body, mind and spirit and calls for a concept of health that embraces the whole in place of the parts, the individual instead of the illness. These ideas have always been central to the philosophies and exercise systems of the East and the Orient – yoga, T'ai Chi, acupuncture and many of the martial arts and Dō-in (pronounced 'doe-in'), an ancient and enlivening body massage.

Common to all these philosophies is a belief in a life force, known as Ki-energy, which is made up of the opposing forces of Yin (negative, female, spiritual) and Yang (positive, male, material). This energy, which has even been photographed (*see note*), is constantly ebbing and flowing. It is when it is well balanced that our physical and spiritual well-being is greatest.

The oriental therapies use different methods to regulate this flow of energy and so restore equilibrium. Dō-in is one of the simplest. It takes just a few minutes to learn and can be practised effectively at home by anyone.

This week's programme
Preliminaries
98 × 1 each leg
115 × 1
98 × 1 each leg
69 × several
34 × 8 each side
110 × 8 each direction
113 until ankles and calves begin to tire
101 3 × 4
59 × 16
83
Active recovery
  cool-down, see page 41
84 × several
103, hands clasped behind head × 3
52 × several
85 until muscles begin to tire
39 × 1
112
Active recovery
  cool-down, see page 41
43, 44, 45 × several
114 × 3 each way
68 × 1

Visual proof of an energy field, or 'aura', emanating from a living body has been given by Kirlian, a Russian scientist. He photographed it by passing an electric current beneath a photographic plate on which the body, or part of the body, is resting. The result was an eerie photograph in which the energy could be seen as a luminous halo. If ailing, the halo is dimmer, though photographs taken before and after spiritual healing sessions have shown increased brightness around the tips of the fingers as the new-found health emanates from the body...

115 ***DŌ-IN*** *Rub hands vigorously together at eye level. Shake them out, clap them together, squeeze and pull each finger out away from you, breathing out strongly. Continue until hands feel warm and fingers tingle. Put hands a little way from each other. Do you feel you are holding an invisible ball of energy? Now you are ready to start.*

a. Lightly rap top of head and brow with knuckles. Rub cheeks and nose, pinch and squeeze eyebrows, rotate eyes, blink vigorously and tap chin with tips of fingers. Now rub ears and pull lobes by letting elbows drop downwards.

b. Interlace fingers and squeeze along sides of neck with heels of hands. Work from base of neck up, breathing out as you press in, in as you release.

c. Cup elbow in hand and make a loose fist with other hand. Pound top of shoulders, working from neck outwards. Start lightly, then rap more vigorously.

d. Breathe in deeply and stretch up. Clench fists loosely and, as you breathe out, thump chest, opening mouth wide and making loud noises.

e. Rap from top of inside arm, to wrist and then up outside of arm . . .

f. Go into flat back, bending from hips. Rap each side of spine, working from head to buttocks.

g. Drop forwards from hips and rap buttocks.

h. Still standing, rap each leg in turn, from top of inner thigh to ankle. Return up outer side.

i. Rub feet vigorously all over, rap along sole of foot from heel to toes, press Achilles tendon and massage area above ankle. Finally massage toes individually, wiggling and rotating each in turn.

Rapping yourself with fists and knuckles may look painful, but it's not at all. The key is to keep hands soft, fists loosely clenched and wrists flexible.

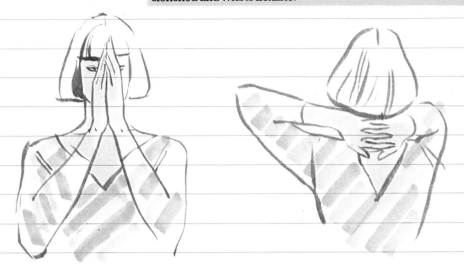

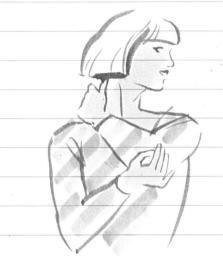

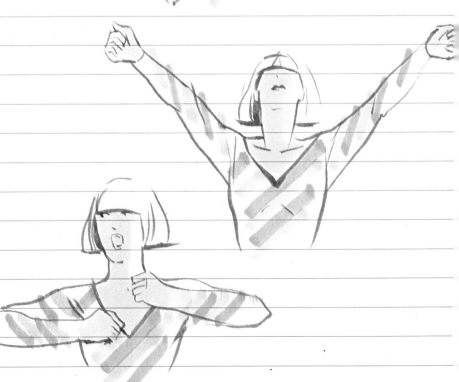

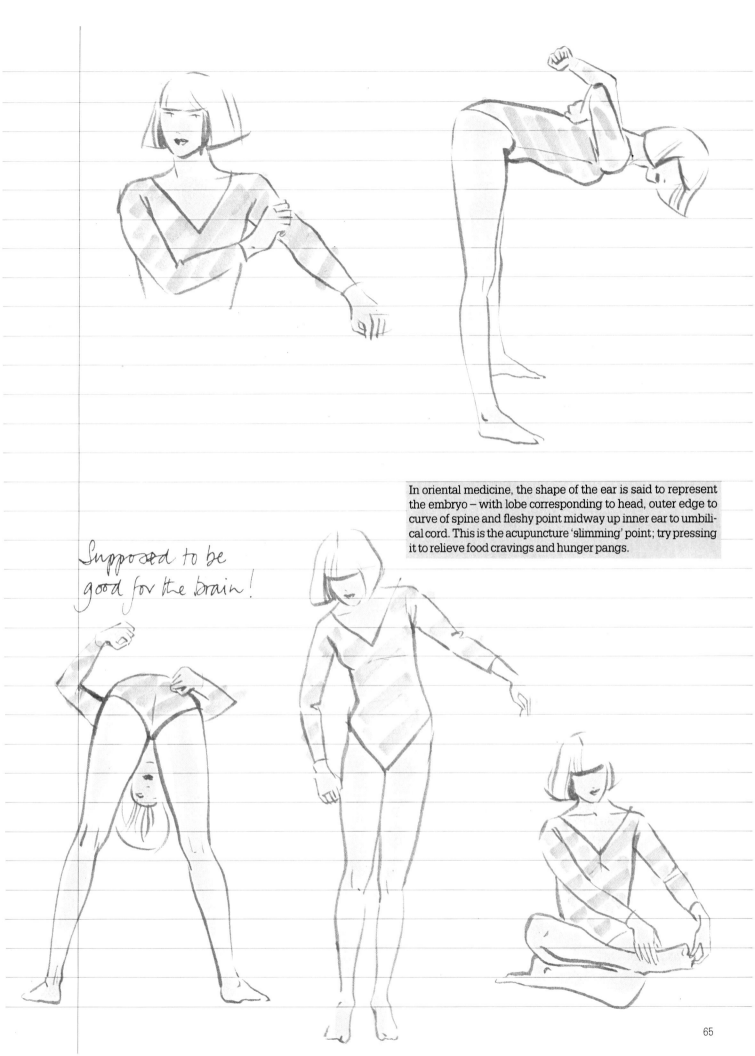

Supposed to be
good for the brain!

In oriental medicine, the shape of the ear is said to represent the embryo – with lobe corresponding to head, outer edge to curve of spine and fleshy point midway up inner ear to umbilical cord. This is the acupuncture 'slimming' point; try pressing it to relieve food cravings and hunger pangs.

WEEK 17: YOGA SUN SALUTATION

Yoga is not so much a form of exercise as a complete philosophy which aims to bring body and mind into close harmony through the practice of postures (*asanas*) and breathing control (*pranayama*). This communion of mind and body takes a lifetime to achieve and is obviously beyond the scope of any book.

Although advanced yoga postures and breathing techniques should be taught by a qualified teacher, the simpler postures, such as those given here, can be practised quite safely by anyone. They will free tension, improve flexibility and give you more joy and confidence in your body.

You don't have to put yourself into bizarre positions or tie yourself into a pretzel to do yoga. Greater freedom and ease of movement is the aim and this comes with practice. If a position feels strained or painful, you are either not doing it properly or are not yet ready to do it. The challenge is to move your body just a little more freely and easily each time.

This week's programme
Preliminaries
116 × 3
34 × 8 each side
110 × 8 each direction
101 3 × 4
59 × 16
83
Active recovery
   cool-down, see page 41
84 × several
103, hands clasped
   behind head × 4
52 × several
85 × 1
39 until muscles begin to
   tire
112
Active recovery
   cool-down, see page 41
66, with weights and
   straight legs × 8 each
   leg
43, 44, 45 × several
114 × 3 each way
58

116 SUN SALUTATION

a. Stand with feet together and palms of hands joined in prayer position. Lengthen up spine and drop shoulders away from ears. Breathe easily in and out several times. Imagine the sun's energy pouring in, filling you with strength and vitality.
b. Breathe in deeply as you reach up with arms. Enjoy feeling of lift and maintain it as you continue to stretch backwards.
c. As you breathe out, bend forwards from hips going smoothly through flat back position until

This sequence stretches all the major muscle groups of the body. Practise first thing in the morning to prepare for the day ahead and later on as a preliminary to any type of vigorous activity or simply to refresh and reinvigorate...

To begin with, the sequence may seem complicated, especially the breathing. But once familiar with it, you will find each movement flows easily into the next.

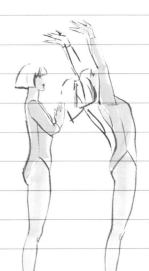
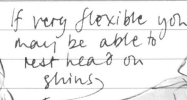

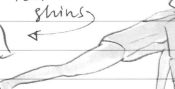

If very flexible you may be able to rest head on shins

hands are flat beside feet, or at least touching floor. Keep legs straight.

d. Breathe in and extend right leg back so that it is fully extended with heel pointing towards back of room. Keep head up and look straight ahead. Your body should now make a straight line from heel of back foot to shoulders.

e. Breathe normally as you take left foot back and place it beside right. You are now in full press-up position (good preparation for week 24). Your back should be flat with no arching or sagging and pelvis tucked under.

f. Breathe in. As you breathe out, lower body so that toes, knees, chest, palms and forehead are all resting on floor. Pelvis should be raised off floor and hands should be as before, with elbows bent and arms by sides.

g. Breathe in. As you breathe out, release position and lie extended on floor with hands by head.

h. Bring hands up to shoulder level and breathe in as you raise head and chest, keeping pelvis flat on floor. Arch head back as you straighten arms.

i. Breathe out and raise hips to form an inverted V, with feet flat on floor and legs straight. Look at toes.

j. Breathe normally as you bring right foot forwards. Keep left foot back and fully extended, resting on toes.

k. Breathe in. As you breathe out, bring left leg up. Place feet together and straighten legs.

l. Breathe in as you straighten up from hips. Bring arms up, lengthening up spine, and then stretch backwards.

m. Breathe out and straighten. Bring hands back to prayer position. Practise whole exercise 3 times in a good rhythm.

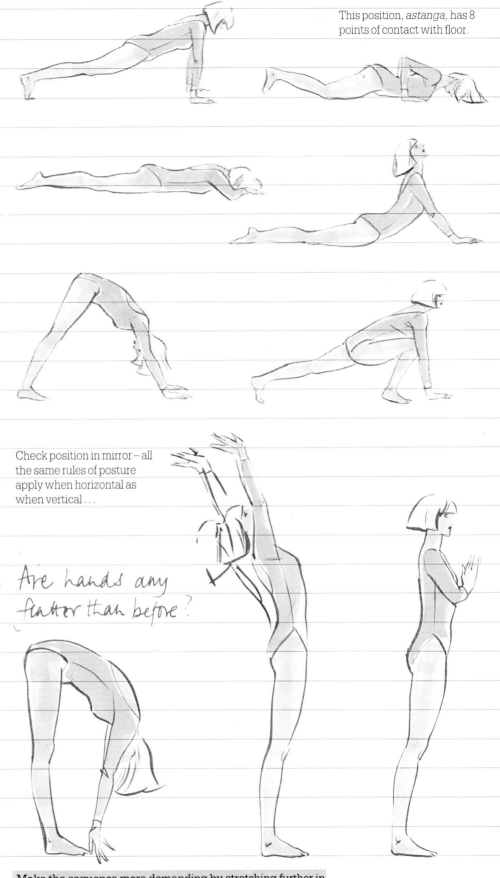

This position, *astanga*, has 8 points of contact with floor.

Check position in mirror – all the same rules of posture apply when horizontal as when vertical...

Are hands any flatter than before?

Make the sequence more demanding by stretching further in each position, using out-breaths to help you. For a greater challenge still, take up Iyengar yoga. Iyengar, one of the great yoga masters, has developed a series of strong sustained stretches to overcome stiffness, help free the body.

67

WEEK 18: SEXUALITY

Sexuality is a quality we can all develop by becoming more aware, more confident, and by using our bodies more fully.

It was the psychologist Wilhelm Reich (1897-1977) who first suggested that mind and body can influence each other in such a way as to interfere with, or to enhance, sexual pleasure. Emotional disturbances, he said, lead to muscular 'blocks' that dam up biological energy and interfere with our capacity for giving and receiving pleasure. Reich called these blocks 'dead zones' because they are the opposite of the sexual impulse which is about being alive in its fullest, most enjoyable sense.

Most of us have dead zones in our bodies – and sometimes in our minds too. Help awaken them with long, slow stretching, specific strengtheners that call on underused muscles and some Feldenkrais work that will enhance awareness by focusing attention on your body.

This week's programme
Preliminaries
116 × 1 slowly, breathing well
43, 44, 45 × several
42 × 1
117 × 1
56 × 1
118 × several
34 × 8 each side
110 × 8 each direction
101 3 × 4
59 × 16
83
Active recovery
  cool-down, see page 41
84 × several
103, hands clasped behind head × 4
52 × several
85, until muscles begin to tire
64 × several
106 × 16 with each ball
112
Active recovery
  cool-down, see page 41
114 × 3 each way
58
N.B. Also this week, pelvic floor exercises **119**, see note

'Sexuality and anxiety are functions of the living organism, operating in opposite directions: pleasurable expansion and anxious contraction...'
Wilhelm Reich *The Function of the Orgasm*

The pelvis can be a major dead zone. The Feldenkrais clock sequence should have helped you gain awareness and mobility there but if you still find it stiff and unresponsive, use your breathing to help you. Lying down, breathe out slowly and deeply and see how your pelvis starts to roll naturally forwards in a continuous forward curve. Reich maintained that this undulatory movement is the position of 'surrender' in which blocked energy is released and that it is the only position in which orgasm can take place.

117 AWARENESS

Lie on back with knees bent and feet flat on floor. Visualize your anus, picturing it as a circle, and squeeze it several times. Now visualize your bladder, picturing it as a tube, and squeeze that several times. Can you differentiate between them? Practise squeezing anus, then bladder, quite hard several times and then go back to squeezing anus softly. Do you notice a difference? Visualizing both anus and bladder together, squeeze them simultaneously. Rest a moment, then squeeze them separately several times. Are you finding it easier to move them independently? If not, continue practising a few times each day until you do...

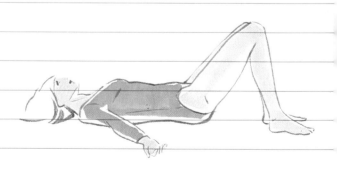

118 **PELVIS** *Standing with feet apart, hands on hips and knees slightly bent, rock pelvis back and forth several times. Then rock it from side to side. Finish with some complete rotations, clockwise and anti-clockwise, making sure that movement is coming from pelvis and not from thighs.*

Are you very stiff? You will get much more supple with practice . . .

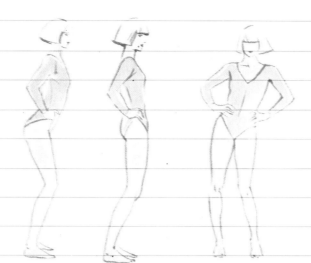

VARIATION . . . Try a figure-of-eight: circle right hip clockwise in a complete rotation; coming through centre, circle left hip anti-clockwise in a complete rotation. Do several then change direction.

The more you use and move your pelvis, the more you will become aware of it as your centre of gravity and balance.

119 **PELVIC FLOOR** *Locate pelvic floor muscles (see note) by trying to stop the flow of urine when you go to the lavatory. Once you have got the feeling, practise contracting and releasing them. Then try contracting them in stages: up one level; pause; up a little more; pause; all the way up; hold and release. Repeat 10 times slowly, then more quickly, several times a day.*

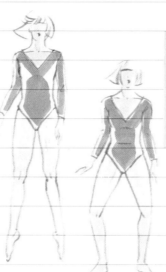

The muscles of the pelvic floor lie like the interconnecting circles of a figure-of-eight around the vagina and urethra (which leads to the bladder) and the anus. Although fundamental to pleasure and sensitivity when making love, few of us even realize where they are much less think of exercising them to keep them firm and strong. This week's exercises not only test their strength but your ability to differentiate between them . . .

Your partner will be able to tell whether you are doing this correctly if he can feel muscles tightening when you make love . . .

Finish with a test: can you jump up and down, legs wide apart as shown, coughing out as you do so without letting urine escape from the bladder? If so, your pelvic floor muscles are in good shape.

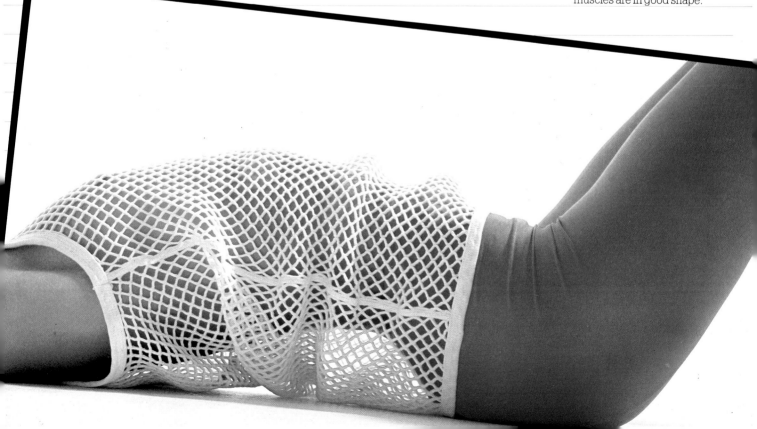

WEEK 19: ROCK AND ROLL

Free-moving, fun, fast and extremely energetic, rock and roll may look easy and carefree but it demands perfect-timing, good coordination, considerable strength, stamina and mobility (particularly in the ankles, hence exercise 121), and a lot of practice to get the footwork right. Start rehearsing today with the specially choreographed rock and roll sequences on page 88. Learn a new section, step by step, each day and you will have mastered the complete sequence by the end of the week...

This week's programme
Preliminaries
32 × several
69 × several
53 × several
120 × 8 each side
121 × 16 each position
113 until ankles and calves begin to tire
101 4 × 4
59 × 16
122
Active recovery
   cool-down, see page 41
84 × several
103, hands clasped behind head × 5
52 × several
85 until muscles begin to tire
Rock and roll practice (see page 88)
112
Active recovery
   cool-down, see page 41
123 × 4
114 × 3 each way
68 × 1

120 **WAIST** *Stand with feet well apart and parallel, hands on chest as shown. Turn torso to right, to back and to centre again rocking body 3 times as you go. Repeat to other side. Practise 8 times each side.*

Rock and roll, the phenomenon of the 50s, seemed to arrive out of nowhere... but in fact it can be traced back as far as West African tribal dancing and, more directly, to the many dance crazes that swept the USA in the 20s and 30s when big bands and glittering ballrooms made dancing available to everyone. Rock and roll borrowed heavily from these crazes before adding some uptempo steps of its own...

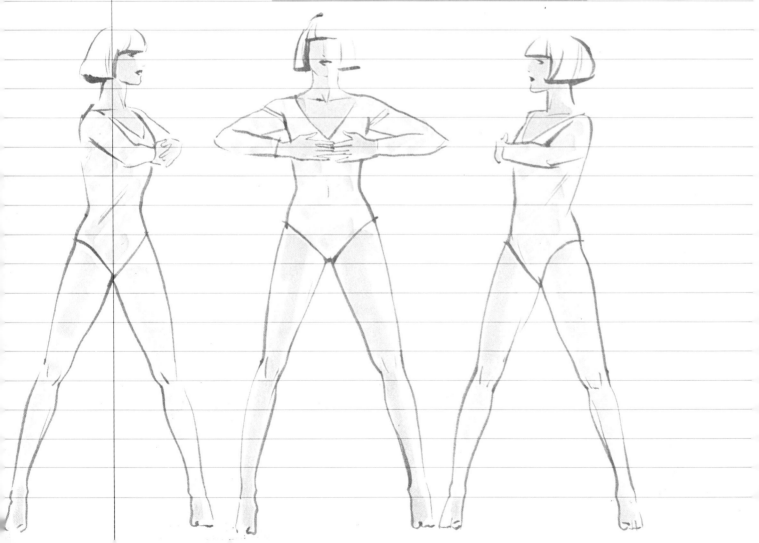

121 LEGS AND ANKLES
Stand well with feet together. Bend knees and lift up onto balls of feet. Straighten legs and return to starting position. Repeat 16 times; then try the same exercise with legs apart; with right leg in front of left; with left leg in front of right.

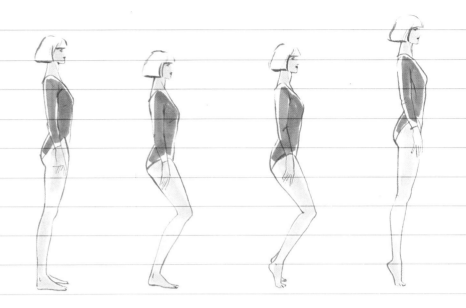

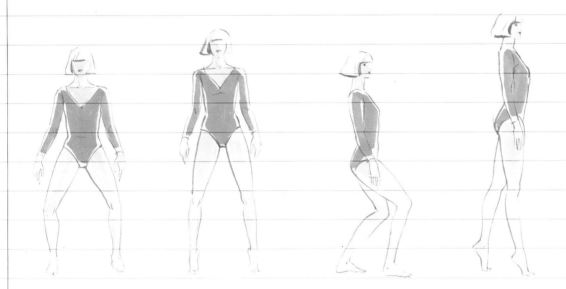

In the mood... Try doing the new exercises, and the aerobic sequence, to one of the rock and roll music suggestions on page 88.

122 LEGS
Stretch one leg back, the other forwards, and place hands on floor. Bounce hips towards floor for 7 counts. Then bring back leg in and bounce knees together for 3 counts. Change legs and repeat. Alternate in this way twice and then stretch one leg back, place its opposite elbow on floor and bounce hips down towards floor as before. Change legs and repeat. Practise twice.

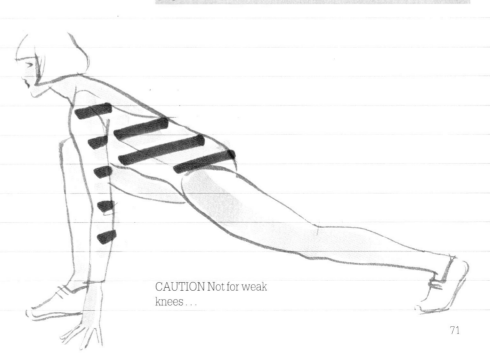

CAUTION Not for weak knees...

123 **WAIST AND INNER THIGHS** *Sit with legs apart, arms outstretched at shoulder level. Lift one arm up over head and stretch over towards opposite foot,* *maintaining length in spine. Return to centre, change arms and repeat to other side. Then reach forwards from hips feeling strong stretch in thighs as you go. Keep back straight. Repeat 3 times.*

VARIATION Try
flexing feet

WEEK 20: MEDITATION

Meditation seems strange to many western minds, but the ability to put all activity aside and to find one's centre again is more important than ever in the rush and tumble of the western lifestyle where time to contemplate, to be passive and to *let* rather than *make* things happen is hardly ever on the schedule.

You don't need a guru or collection of Sanskrit words in order to meditate, just a mind that is open, receptive, willing to see what happens. Don't you owe it to yourself to find out why so many people become calmer and happier once they start meditating regularly? Follow the simple directions *below*.

This week's programme
Preliminaries
20-minute meditation practice
124 or **125**
56 × 1
57 × 3 minutes each foot
116 × 1, breathing well
110 × 8 each direction
120 × 8 each side
59 × 16
122
Active recovery cool-down, see page 41
103, hands clasped behind head × 5
52 × several
85 until muscles begin to tire
123 × 4
112
Active recovery cool-down, see page 41
42 × 1
81 × 1
117 × 1
58
124 or **125**

'...that serene and blessed mood,
In which the affections gently lead us on –
Until, the breath of this corporeal frame
And even the motion of our human blood,
Almost suspended, we are laid asleep
In body, and become a living soul:
While with an eye made quiet by the power
Of harmony, and the deep power of joy,
We see into the life of things...'
William Wordsworth. *Lines composed a few miles above Tintern Abbey*

Three requirements for meditation:

1. No distractions. Meditate in a quiet place. Take a watch to check on time occasionally but not an alarm.

2. Comfort. Don't lie down – it's too easy to go to sleep; sit instead with spine straight and supported by cushions if necessary.

3. No judgements. Don't expect too much right away. Instead of being preoccupied with how well you are doing, adopt a calm, passive, non-judging attitude and simply enjoy the peace of quiet contemplation.

124 MEDITATION I

Sit with spine straight and legs out in front of you. Now bend one knee and place foot high on opposite thigh, then either lift second leg over first or tuck it beneath in half lotus or sit in simple cross-legs if neither position is comfortable. Place hands on knees, close eyes, relax body, soften face and turn attention inwards. You now need something to meditate on. Here are two alternatives. Practise both and continue with the one that you find works best.

Breathing. The important thing for this is to be aware only of the breath as it comes and goes. If other thoughts drift in, do not let them intervene; allow them to pass on. Starting on an out-breath, count each breath until you reach 10. If random thoughts rush in, go back to the beginning and start all over again. With practice, your concentration will improve.

The lotus position *padmasana*, the position of enlightenment, symbolizes our own spiritual nature with our roots in the mud, our stem rising through the water in search of light and our head blossoming in the clarity of self-realization...

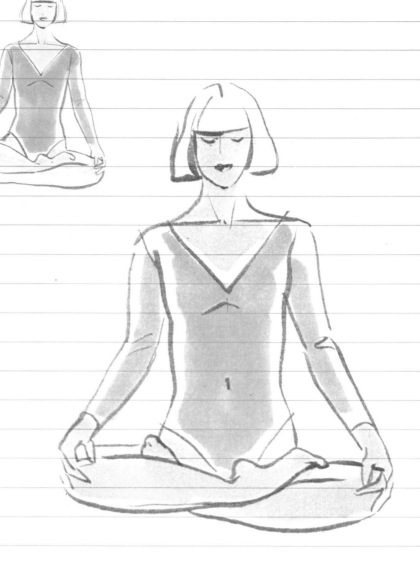

125 MEDITATION II

Sitting as above, and being lightly aware of your breathing, repeat a single syllable word on each out-breath, silently or out loud. You might like to choose a word yourself, or use a Sanskrit 'mantra' such as the Siddha 'OM' (pronounced 'Oh-m'). Or try the word 'ONE' recommended by Herbert Benson in The Relaxation Response. *Whichever you choose, allow your mind to dwell on it maintaining an attitude of passive, relaxed concentration.*

When the eyes are active, the brain is active too. If thoughts rush in while meditating, soften your eyes and you will find your mind becomes still again.

Breathing is a useful path to meditation because it is a bridge between the voluntary and the involuntary, the conscious and the unconscious. 'The mind rides the breath' is how the eastern gurus put it.

Breathing out is the breath of surrender, of letting go. When we expire, we die and release our hold on life; when we give birth the exhalation expels the baby; when we have an orgasm, we gasp; when we breathe out in meditation we surrender the self to greater consciousness. The Mahayama Buddhists in Tibet, in an extension of this practice, breathe in the suffering of others in the form of visualized black smoke and breathe out love and compassion in the form of a white light to heal and to bless.

WEEK 21: BASIC BALLET

The exacting standards of classical ballet are such that to be good you have to start young – not just because of the years of training required but also because its strict disciplines shape the body in a certain way. Happily, though, there is still much to be gained from ballet, such as improved strength and an enjoyable feeling of grace and renewed control over your body, without having to reach the great technical heights demanded of the classical dancer.

Many basic ballet movements make useful general exercises. They demand good control, correct technique and suppleness at certain joints – in particular the hips where the 'turn out' (rotation of the hip in the joint) is considered paramount. Strength, too, is important. The slight willowy shape of the classical dancer belies tremendous power, particularly in the legs and feet...

This week's programme
Preliminaries
116 × 2
126 × 4 each side
127 × 8 each side
128 × 4 each side
129 × 8
130 × 8 each side
131 × 8 each side
132 × 8 each side
110 × 8 each side
123 × 4
101 4 × 4
59 × 16
112
Active recovery cool-down, see page 41
103, hands clasped behind head × 5
52 × several
85, add 0.5 kg (1 lb) weight to each ankle until muscles begin to tire
114 × 3 each way
133
Active recovery cool-down, see page 41
43, 44, 45 × several
58

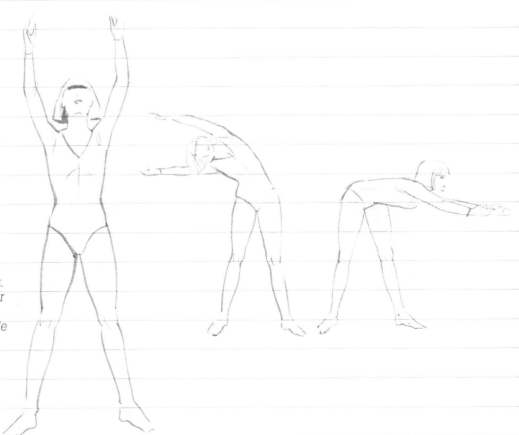

126 WARM-UP *Stand in second position (feet apart and turned out) with arms raised to ceiling. Bend over to right, bringing arms and head over too. Then twist into diagonal forward stretch, with flat back, and move round to opposite corner keeping hips level throughout. Now twist again so you stretch to left. Return to centre and lower arms to shoulder level. Repeat 3 times to each side in a nice easy rhythm.*

127 TENDU *Stand well in first position (heels together, toes out, arms and hands as shown), with pelvis tucked under and spine lengthened. Extend leg to side, brushing foot along floor until toes are fully pointed. Keep body centered and both legs straight. Practise 8 times; then change legs and repeat to other side.*

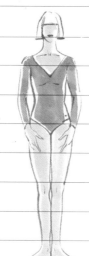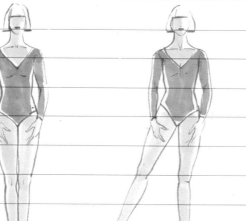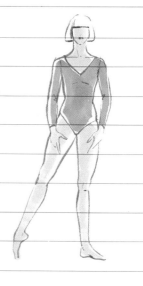

Leg turns out from hip in first position – one of the most basic ballet stances.

Preliminary to *battement* leg-raising exercises . . .

BONUS Good for balance.

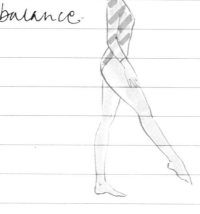

Keep supporting leg straight throughout

128 PETITS BATTEMENTS *Stand well with feet together. Brush one foot forwards along floor and up, pointing toes, to height shown here. Repeat to side, back and to side again. Make sure you keep body centered, hips level and back vertical throughout. Practise 4 times with each foot and then repeat whole exercise, but this time flex and point foot 4 times each time you lift it.*

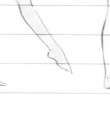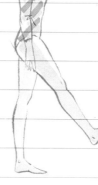

BONUS Good for balance.

129 DEVELOPPÉ *Stand well with feet together, arms at shoulder level. Lift one leg so thigh is parallel to floor and hips are level. Extend leg forwards, pointing toe, in one slow controlled movement. Your whole leg should now be parallel to floor. Lower to tendu and bring feet together. Practise 8 times; then change legs and repeat exercise.*

The more you lift knee the higher leg will go

Ballet is not a complete form of exercise: upper body loses out to lower body and suppleness to strength. So, if you want to use it as a means of keeping fit, complement with some good general stretches, plenty of flexibility work on shoulders and spine (the twists in particular) and strengtheners for the upper body.

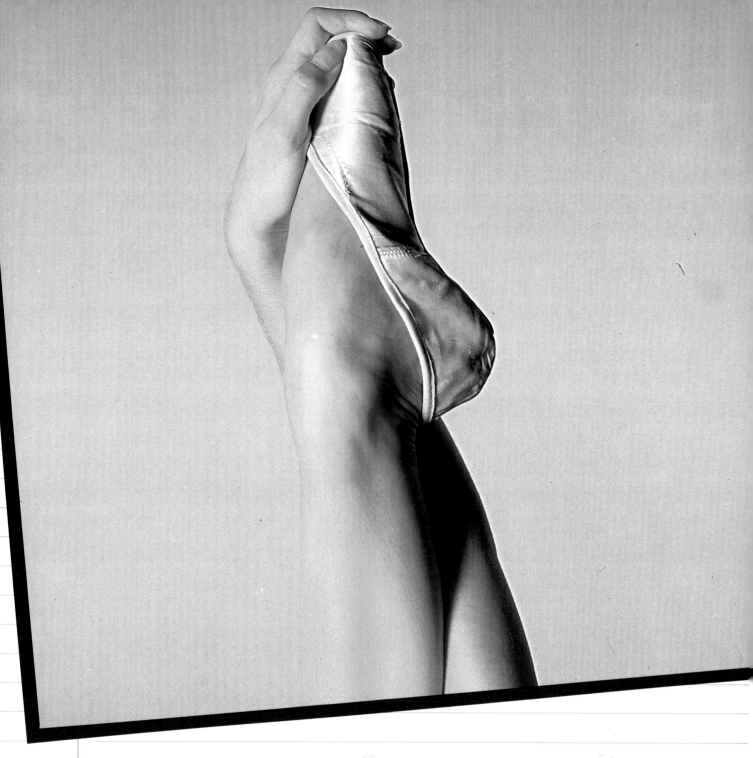

130 DEVELOPPÉ À LA SECONDE

Stand well in first position with arms at shoulder level. Lift one leg so toes are by inside of other knee and extend out to side. Practise 8 times, in a slow controlled manner; then change legs and repeat. Now try it again, but this time extend leg forwards instead of sideways keeping heel to the side to practise turn out.

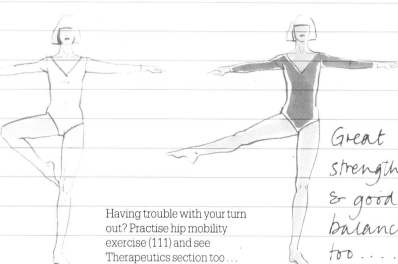

Having trouble with your turn out? Practise hip mobility exercise (111) and see Therapeutics section too . . .

Great strengthener & good for balance too . . . .

131 EPAULEMENTS

Stand in second position with arms at shoulder level. Press one shoulder forwards and down. Then repeat to other side, feeling connection between shoulders as you do so. Practise 8 times each side and then repeat exercise walking forwards, one step at a time, bringing each shoulder forwards with its opposite leg.

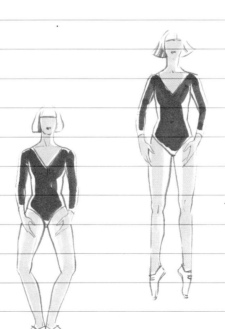

132 RETIRÉ

Stand in first position with arms at shoulder level. Lift one leg up until thigh is parallel to floor and place foot up inside of supporting leg so toes touch knee. Return to starting position. Practise 8 times each side.

keep supporting leg straight throughout

133 JUMPS

Extend your freestyle sequence by 1 minute, adding any movements you enjoy and these ballet jumps. Stand in first position with arms as shown, bend knees in demi plié and spring up into air, pointing toes. Land lightly, bending knees in demi plié again, and spring up again, feeling leg muscles tighten. Be sure to keep pelvis tucked under and back vertical.

CAUTION Failing to bend knees may jar spine.

Helps you to think 'up' as well as 'forward' when you move

WEEK 22: BARRE WORK

Here are a few more basic ballet movements using a barre to help you balance. Look on it as an aid, not a leaning post, and hold onto it lightly with the tips of the fingers. If you place too much weight on it, the line of your body will be wrong and the exercise less effective. If you do not have a barre, use the back of a chair – a good substitute because you will know you are not using it properly if it starts tipping or lifting.

Thigh muscles work hard to maintain stability when doing pliés. If you find them difficult, or your knee hurts, only go as far as comfortable and if pain is felt, STOP.

This week's programme
Preliminaries
116 × 2
134 × 4
135 × 4
136 × 4
137 × 4
128, progression **138** × 4 each side
132 on demi-pointe, hand resting lightly on barre × 8 each side
139 × 8
110 × 8 each direction in sets of 2 each time
101 4 × 5
59 × 16
122
Active recovery cool-down, see page 41
103, hands clasped behind head × 5
52 × several
85, with weight until muscles begin to tire
140 × 4 each side
5-minute freestyle aerobic sequence
Active recovery cool-down, see page 41
39 × 1
43, 44, 45 × several
58

134 DEMI PLIÉ
Stand in first position, holding barre as shown, with spine lengthened and pelvis centered. Maintaining upright posture, bend knees so that they go directly over feet. Bend them as far as you can without lifting heels off floor for 2 counts. Return to starting position, fully extending legs, for 2 counts. Repeat 3 times.

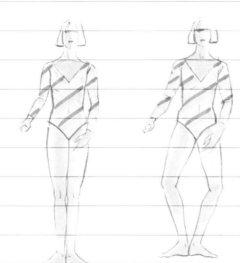

Never force first position – turn out will improve as hips become more mobile

135 GRAND PLIÉ
Standing in first position, as before, with spine well lifted and buttocks tucked under, pass through demi plié position to a turned-out squatting position, lifting heels from floor, for 4 counts. Press heels down and return to starting position for 4 counts. Don't fall forwards. Repeat 3 times.

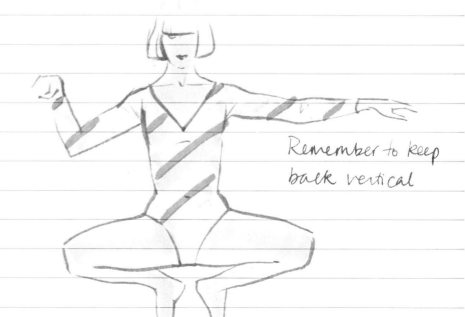

Remember to keep back vertical

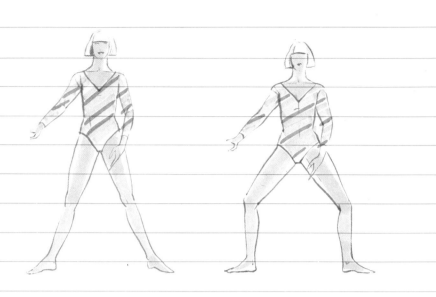

136 **DEMI PLIÉ** *Stand in second position and bend knees over toes as you go into a demi plié for 2 counts, keeping spine straight, buttocks tucked under and feet flat on floor. Return to starting position for 2 counts. Repeat 3 times.*

137 **GRAND PLIÉ**
Standing in second position, pass through demi plié and go down as far as you can without lifting heels for 4 counts. Return to starting position for 4 counts. Repeat 3 times.

CAUTION If knees hurt, stop and turn to Therapeutics exercises on page 123.

Pliés, the opening exercises in the ballet class routine, warm up muscles, loosen joints, promote strength and improve balance. Once you have mastered them at the barre, try them in the centre of the room...

138 **PETITS BATTEMENTS**
Use barre for this progression of exercise 128. As you lift foot off floor rise onto demi-point (ball of supporting foot) and lower gradually as you return to starting position. Repeat to side, to back and to side again keeping back vertical as before. Practise exercise 4 times each side; then try flex/point variation.

The principles of good posture apply as much as ever at the barre. Keep weight evenly balanced, spine lengthened, pelvis centered and buttocks tucked under – especially when doing pliés where benefits to be gained depend on doing them correctly...

139 BALANCE

Stand in second position away from barre, with arms at shoulder level. Raise arms gracefully above head, as shown, as you rise up on demi-points, keeping legs fully extended. Slowly lower heels to ground. Repeat 7 times.

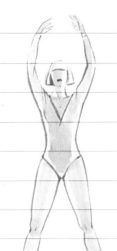

Be careful not to tip forwards as you rise

140 WAIST

Place one leg on barre and raise arms above head. Breathe in. As you breathe out, stretch sideways away from barre as far as is comfortable, feeling a good stretch along side for 4 counts. Return to centre for 4 counts and then repeat stretch to other side. Practise 4 times each side.

Height of barre or chair back should be such that raised leg is parallel to ground as here

Not a classical ballet movement but a great stretch on way down, and a good strengthener on way up too . . .

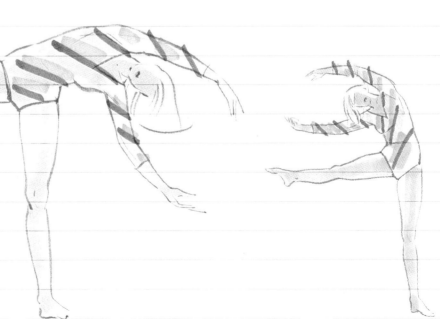

WEEK 23: JAZZ

Easy to recognize, almost impossible to describe, jazz has always escaped strict definition. With individuality and freedom the keynotes, there are as many different styles and interpretations as performers. In some, it's the isolation of rib and hip that's important, in others the swing, in yet others the 'jazzed-up' Latin-American dance steps of the samba and rumba.

In their efforts to break free from the strict, disciplines of classical ballet, both jazz and contemporary dance have remained deliberately loose. You will feel the difference as soon as you start this week's warm-up. Once you have mastered the routine on pages 92-7, start improvising. Add a swing in the hips, make the movements more expressive, mix them up to create new combinations or even invent some of your own... That's the essence of jazz.

This week's programme

Preliminaries
32 × several
141 × several
53 × several
142 × 4 each way
143 × 4 each way
144 × 8
123 × 4
101 4 × 5
59 × 16
122
Active recovery
  cool-down, see page 41
103, hands clasped
  behind head × 5
52 × several
85, with weight until
  muscles begin to tire
75 × up to 8
Jazz practice (see page
  92)
5-minute freestyle
  aerobic sequence
  including 145 and **146**,
  × 8 each side
Active recovery
  cool-down, see page 41
43, 44, 45 × several
58

Unlike the highly-organized disciplines of classical ballet and ballet music, which are strictly notated and choreographed down to the last note or step, jazz dance and jazz music rely as much on spontaneity and improvisation as they do on a written score. And there is another difference: in classical music and ballet everything happens on the beat; in jazz the accent of the rhythm is more often syncopated – i.e. more likely to be off the beat than on it.

Hands are very important and often used with palms facing forwards and fingers spread ('jazz palms') to initiate, emphasize or finish a movement.

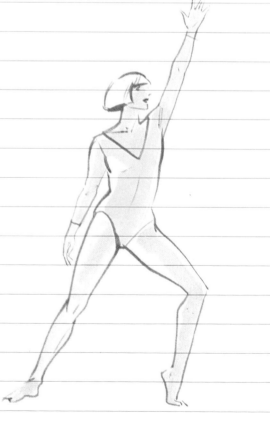

141 **SIDES** *This jazzed-up version of the side lunge and upward stretch (69) works as a good warm-up and will also help you with your timing. Stand with feet 60 cm (2 ft) apart and slightly turned out. Lunge onto right leg lifting right arm to ceiling, palm facing front, for a really good stretch. Repeat to left. Start by stretching to each side* *for 8 counts, then 4 counts, then 2 counts, then 1 count. Remember to count up to 8 twice through at each stage, so that you are stretching twice to each side to begin with, 8 times to each side to finish. Now run through the exercise again, lifting your heel off the ground but still stretching as far as possible to each side.*

Once you've got the idea, try it to music

82

142 **HIPS** *Stand with feet hip-width apart and parallel. Bend knees and tilt hips up and forwards, then back to centre, then to back. Now try it again but this time move hips forwards and back, passing smoothly through the centre each time.*

Starting with hips well centered again, move them to right, to centre, to left and back to centre. Then move them straight through from right to left, passing smoothly through the centre each time.

Now try a square: tilt hips forwards, to right, to back, to left and forwards again before finishing back in the centre. Practise in both directions.

Finish with a circle: tilt hips forwards, then curve them to left, to back, to right and forwards again. Return to the centre and reverse the movement.

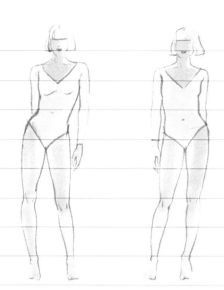

Isolations, one of the signature movements of classical jazz, aim to get ribcage and hips moving independently of each other. At first, only small movements may be possible, but persevere. You will become more supple with practice...

143 **RIBCAGE** *Stand well with feet hip-width apart, arms by sides, spine lengthened and ribcage lifted.*

Now move ribcage forwards over hips, then to centre, then to back; then, lifting ribcage as before, move it forwards and back, passing smoothly through centre each time.

Lift ribcage again and move it to right, to centre, and to left; then move it to right and left, passing smoothly through centre each time you change.

Now try making a square: lift ribcage and move it forwards, then to left, then back, then to right, then forwards and, finally, back to centre. Try it in other direction too.

Finish with a circle: lift ribcage and move it forwards, then round to right, lthen to back, then round to left, then forwards again before coming back to centre. Try it in both directions.

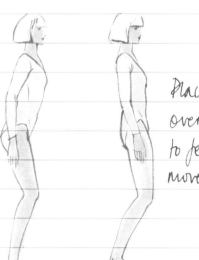

Place hands over ribs to feel movement

144 **BALANCE** *Try this jazz version of last week's exercise. Standing in second position, with arms at shoulder level, raise arms upwards so that palms are facing forwards. Now rise up onto balls of feet, keeping legs fully extended, for 2 counts. Lower heels to floor for 2 counts. Practise 8 times. Then repeat whole exercise, raising and lowering heels for 1 count each time.*

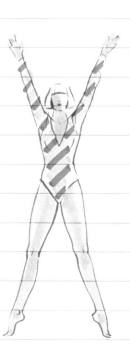

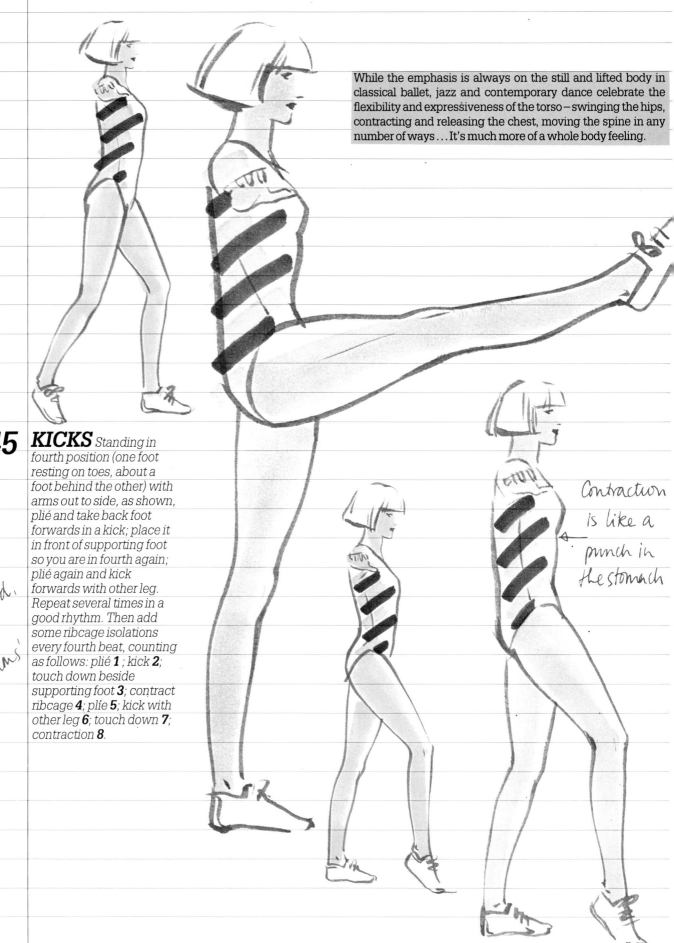

While the emphasis is always on the still and lifted body in classical ballet, jazz and contemporary dance celebrate the flexibility and expressiveness of the torso – swinging the hips, contracting and releasing the chest, moving the spine in any number of ways . . . It's much more of a whole body feeling.

145 **KICKS** *Standing in fourth position (one foot resting on toes, about a foot behind the other) with arms out to side, as shown, plié and take back foot forwards in a kick; place it in front of supporting foot so you are in fourth again; plié again and kick forwards with other leg. Repeat several times in a good rhythm. Then add some ribcage isolations every fourth beat, counting as follows: plié* **1** *; kick* **2***; touch down beside supporting foot* **3***; contract ribcage* **4***; plié* **5***; kick with other leg* **6***; touch down* **7***; contraction* **8***.*

VARIATION = Kick with foot flexed, hands as 'jazz palms'

Contraction is like a punch in the stomach

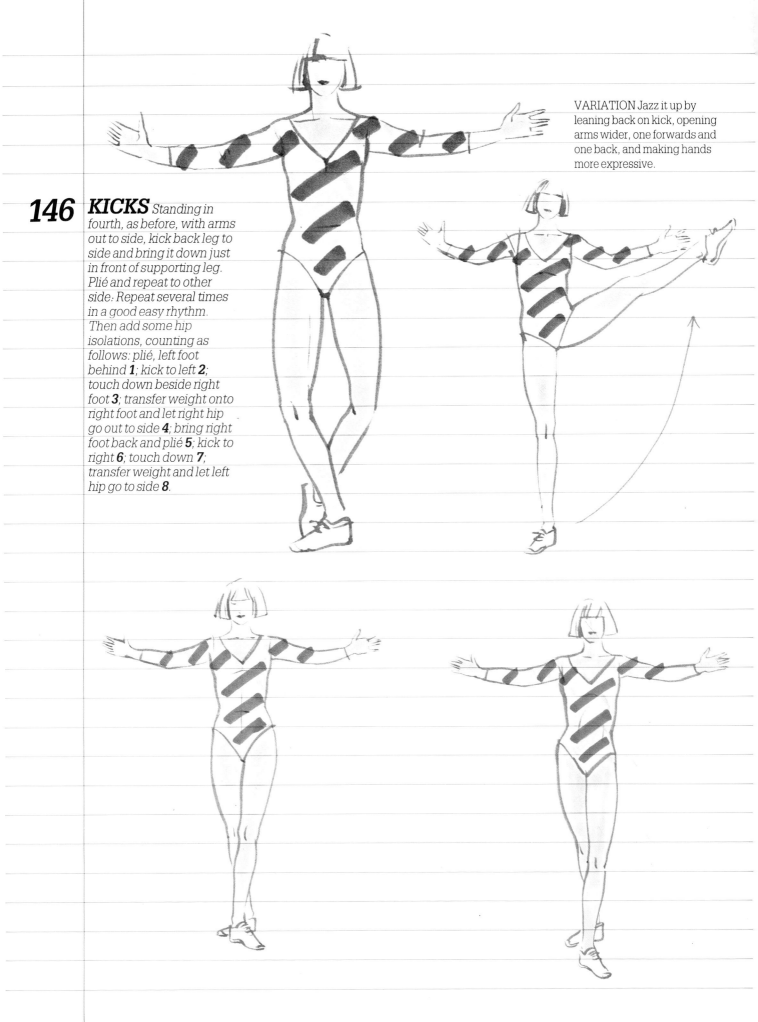

VARIATION Jazz it up by leaning back on kick, opening arms wider, one forwards and one back, and making hands more expressive.

146 | **KICKS** *Standing in fourth, as before, with arms out to side, kick back leg to side and bring it down just in front of supporting leg. Plié and repeat to other side. Repeat several times in a good easy rhythm. Then add some hip isolations, counting as follows: plié, left foot behind **1**; kick to left **2**; touch down beside right foot **3**; transfer weight onto right foot and let right hip go out to side **4**; bring right foot back and plié **5**; kick to right **6**; touch down **7**; transfer weight and let left hip go to side **8**.*

WEEK 24: GRADUATION

Week 24, graduating with honours, and you will be feeling really fit – strong, agile, powerful, swift and in altogether better shape than you have probably been for a long time.

After all this regular exercising, you may now want to have a break, perhaps to take up a new sport or exercise form, such as fencing, yoga or one of the 3 training schedules on pages 98-105. Have the confidence to try anything. Your body is perfectly primed for the challenge.

This week's programme
Preliminaries
116 × 2, breathing well
140 × 4 each side
147 × 3 each side
148 × 4, breathing well
149 × 2 each way
150 × 4 each side
151
Active recovery cool-down, see page 41
84 × several
103, hands behind head holding 0.5 kg/(1 lb) weight, work up to 5
52 × several
85 with 1 kg/(2 lb) weight on each ankle until muscles begin to tire
152 × up to 20
6-minute freestyle aerobic sequence OR **Rock and roll/Jazz routine**
Active recovery cool down, see page 41
39, aiming to rest head on legs with back flat × 1
43, 44, 45 × several
58
124

147 CROUCH

Standing with feet about 60 cm (2 ft) apart, do a small pelvic tilt and lift up onto toes, bringing arms out to balance. Bend knees and twist slowly to side and then round to the back, dropping leading arm to touch far ankle. Return to front equally slowly. Repeat 4 times smoothly to each side.

BONUS Excellent for balance

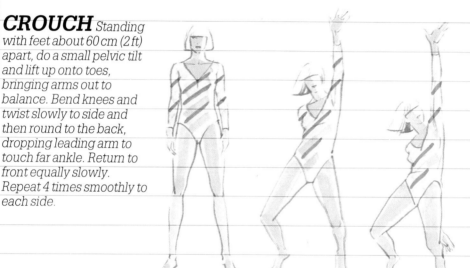

To finish, a super-class to help maintain fitness, and a few more demanding exercises. Try them and, for future weeks, change the programme to incorporate earlier exercises you found helpful. Good luck!

148 ARMS

Sitting cross-legged in your non-habitual way (remember week 4, exercise 40?), with spine lengthened and chest lifted, raise arms above head and cross hands so palms are together. Work arms down towards head, pressing palms together and elbows back. Then work them up again. Cross hands the other way and repeat. Practise exercise twice.

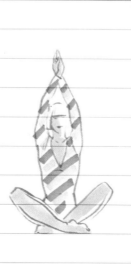

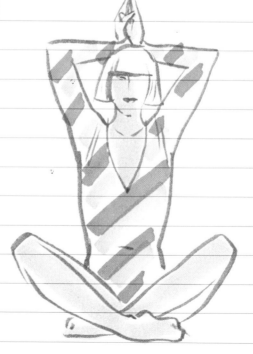

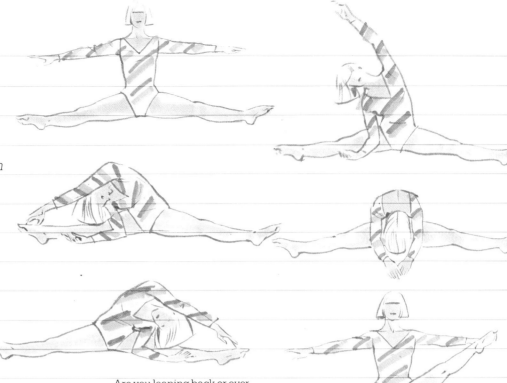

149 **WAIST AND LEGS** *Sit on floor with legs apart and arms out at shoulder level. Lift right arm up, twist and stretch onto left knee. Keeping back flat, continue round in a circle to right knee. As you come back up, raise right leg, without leaning back, so that it is fully extended and naturally turned out. Release and repeat to other side. Work up to 5 repetitions on each side.*

Are you leaning back or over to side when you lift leg? Use a mirror to check or ask someone to watch.

Point foot too, for a different stretch

150 **BACKS OF THIGHS** *Lie on back. Bend one knee and press it into chest for 7 counts. Then extend leg, keeping knee pulled up, and flex foot. Pull leg back, gently but firmly, breathing out for 4 counts. Repeat with other leg. Do 4 times.*

151 **SQUATS** *Now extend your aerobic sequence to 10 minutes and add these side squats. Squat down, place both hands on floor and stretch one leg out to side. Now hop leg back in to meet the other and then stretch other leg out, keeping both hands on floor all the time.*

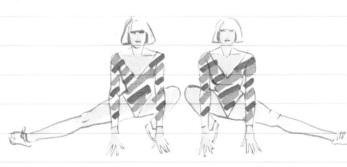

CAUTION Not for weak knees. See Therapeutics section on page 123 instead.

152 **UPPER BODY** *Lie down on your front, hands just under shoulders. Keeping body long and straight, breathe in. As you breathe out, push yourself up, maintaining line in back. Breathe in and lower, without touching floor, and breathe out and push up again. Start with 5 press-ups and work up to 20 in sets of 5.*

Rock and roll

This rock and roll sequence is divided into six sections. Learn one each day and then put them all together on the seventh for the complete dance routine. The *da capo* musical symbol (:‖) at the end of a musical phrase indicates the end of a section. Once you reach it, go right back to the beginning again and practise that part of the sequence again, until you get the steps right. Then put it to music, using one of the suggestions given.

When you get to the lifts (Day 5), bear in mind that these are extended jumps – your partner should never have to support your full weight. Practise several small lifts before aiming for the height shown here.

Music to practise to

Duke's Place by Duke Ellington
In The Mood by Glen Miller
Swing Brother Swing by Count Basie
Rock Around the Clock by Bill Haley

Glossary

Air step any acrobatic movement involving a jump or a lift.
Charleston exuberant dance step from which many of the later ones evolved, involving flicking feet out to either side (partners use opposite feet).
Hip swings an air step in which the woman swings her legs up to one side, resting her hip on his hip, and then to the other without landing inbetween.
Lindy break series of steps used to finish a dance phrase and prepare for the next, usually involving some sort of air step and twist.
Lindy hop a syncopated kick, travelling across the floor, changing legs between each kick.
Straddle split a floor step performed by the man, who balances on one hand and shoots his legs out from underneath him.
The rock the basic rock and roll step, forwards and back holding hands and then changing places.
Through the trenches a stationary step kicking to front, side, back and side again, finishing by jumping with legs apart and then together.

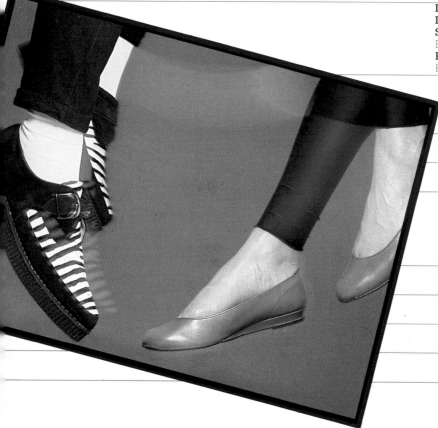

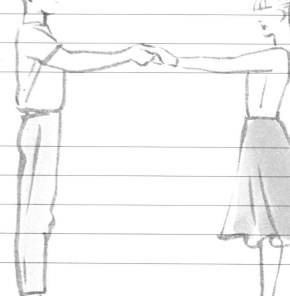

Start facing each other with hands joined, and feet together.

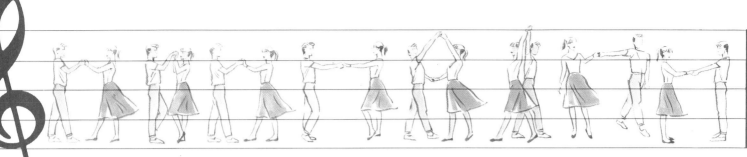

1 Do 'the rock': step forward onto right foot
2 and bring left foot up, lifting heel.
3 Step back with left foot,
4 returning to starting position.

5 Raise arms as shown and change sides
6 by stepping underneath his arm
7 and out to the side, bringing arms down
8 to finish facing each other.

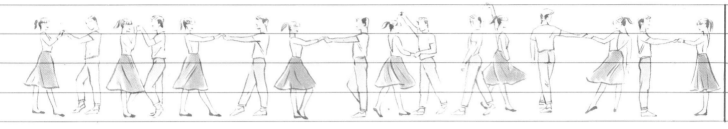

1 Now repeat 'the rock'. Step onto right foot
2 and bring left foot up, lifting heel.
3 Step back with left foot
4 returning to starting position.

5 Raise arms
6 stepping underneath his arm again
7 and to the side. Bring arms down
8 to finish in starting position

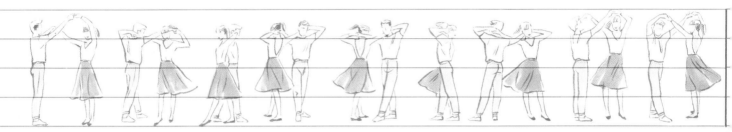

AND Take arms up
1 and, resting them behind head, step round to right
2, 3, 4, 5, 6 for 7 steps, starting with the right foot and

7 bringing arms up on the seventh.
8 Swivel round on the spot to right, through 180 degrees.

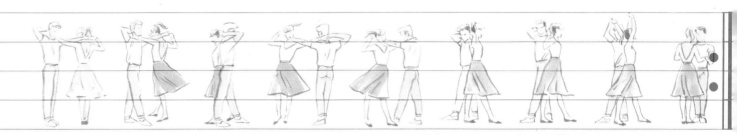

AND Rest arms behind head again
1, 2, 3, 4, 5, 6 and step round to left for 7 steps

7 bringing arms up on the seventh and uncrossing them
8 to finish facing each other.

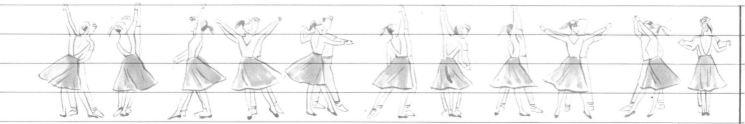

1,2 Stepping to her right (his left), swing arms up.
3,4 Stepping to left, swing arms up.
5 Turn to left, bringing lower arms through
6 and continue turning, through back-to-back position,
7, 8 until facing each other again.

1, 2 Stepping to left (his right), swing arms up.
3, 4 Stepping to right, swing arms up.
5 Turn to left, bring lower arms through
6 and continue turning, through back-to-back position,
7, 8 until facing each other again.

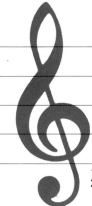
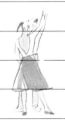
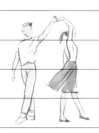
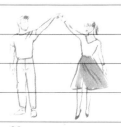
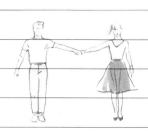

1 Raise arms as shown
2 and step underneath his raised arm, turning towards front.

3 Lower arms
4 and finish side by side.

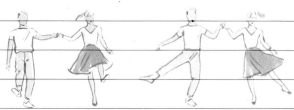
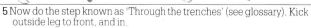
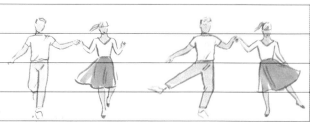

5 Now do the step known as 'Through the trenches' (see glossary). Kick outside leg to front, and in,
6 to side and in,

7 to back, and in,
8 and to side again.

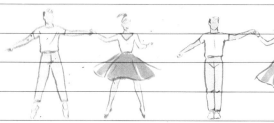
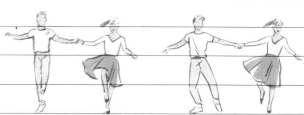

1 Jump feet apart, bending knees,
2 and together again

3 Go 'Through the trenches' again, kicking inside leg to front,
4 to side,

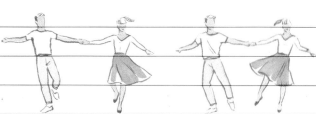
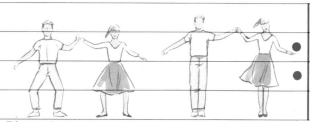

5 to back,
6 and to side again.

7 Jump to feet apart, bending knees
8 and together again.

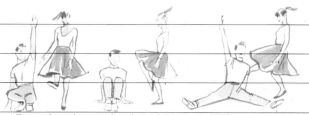
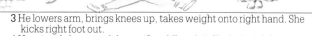

1 Facing front, he crouches down, left arm raised. She does the 'Lindy hop', kicking right foot out.
AND He lowers arm, takes weight onto left hand. She hops onto right foot, starting to travel around him.
2 He raises right arm and does a 'Straddle split'. She kicks left foot out.

3 He lowers arm, brings knees up, takes weight onto right hand. She kicks right foot out.
4 He raises left arm and does a 'Straddle split'. She kicks left foot out.
5 He lowers arm, brings knees up, transfers weight. She kicks right foot out.

DAY 3

90

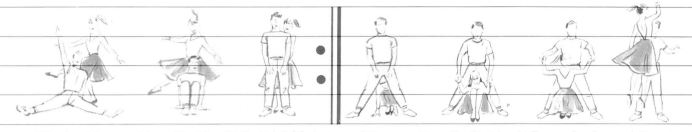

6 He raises right arm and does a 'Straddle split'. She kicks left foot out.
7 He lowers arm, brings knees up, transfers weight. She kicks right foot out.
8 Finish, as shown, with her directly behind him.

DAY 4
1 Change position with a 'Lindy break'. She crouches down and sits on the floor, he reaches for her hands
2 and pulls her through.
3 She squats down and jumps into a turn of 360 degrees,
4 to land in front of him, bending knees.

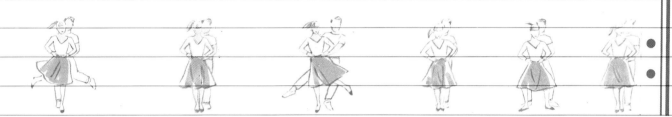

5 With his hands over hers, they do a 'Charleston' – she kicks to right, and he kicks to left –
AND and then, touching down,
6 she kicks to left and he kicks to right,

AND and then, touching down,
7 jump feet apart
8 and together again.

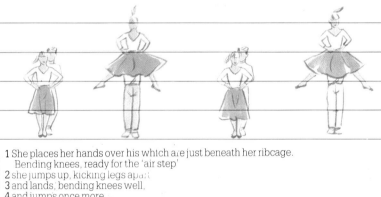

DAY 5
1 She places her hands over his which are just beneath her ribcage. Bending knees, ready for the 'air step'
2 she jumps up, kicking legs apart
3 and lands, bending knees well,
4 and jumps once more

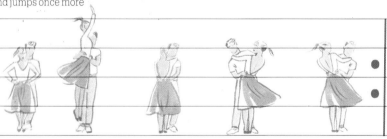

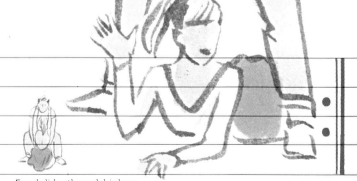

5 and lands again, bending knees,
AND and jumps up, a 'Lindy break', turning through 180 degrees
6 to land facing him with her hands round his neck, his hands on her waist.
7 Peep over each other's shoulders, first to one side
8 then the other.

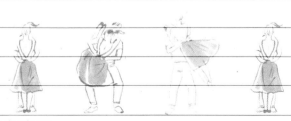

DAY 6
1 Bending knees,
2 she jumps into a 'Hip swing', swinging her legs to one side so her hip and thigh are resting on his hip
3 and then to the other side, without landing in between.
4 Landing in front of him, she bends knees well

5 and slides through his legs
6, 7, 8 to turn on her front. Both wave hands.

Jazz

This jazz sequence, like the rock and roll one on the previous pages, is divided into six sections – with a *da capo* symbol (:||) at the end of each section. Learn one each day and then put the whole routine together on the seventh.

If unfamiliar with jazz and jazz music, start simply by choosing one of the musical options suggested and tap or clap the beat. Once you feel easy with it, take off the music and work out the steps (preferably wearing jazz or other leather-soled shoes). *Then* put music and steps together. When you get the swing of it, incorporate the variations suggested in the text beneath the pictures. Feel free to improvise, too. Learn more by taking classes. These are now offered at many exercise and dance studios.

Glossary

Battement a kick or leg lift.
Epaulement a shoulder movement in which one shoulder is thrust forward and the other back; always performed *in opposition* (see below) with walking step.
Jazz attitude a striking posture in which leg is lifted and held, bent either forwards or back – a jazz equivalent of the classical arabesque.
Jazz palms hands held flexed at wrist so that palms face forwards.
Lay-back leg kicks forwards as torso leans back – a wide, open movement.
Lunge weight transfer forwards, backwards or to one side, bending knee.
Opposition stationary movement or walking step in which shoulder or arm goes forward with opposite foot.
Plié bended knees, usually in preparation for a movement such as a kick.

Music to practise to

Brazilia by John Klemmer
Tropico by Gato Barbieri
Sanborn by David Sanborn
The Shuffle by Kenny G
Rise by Herb Alpert

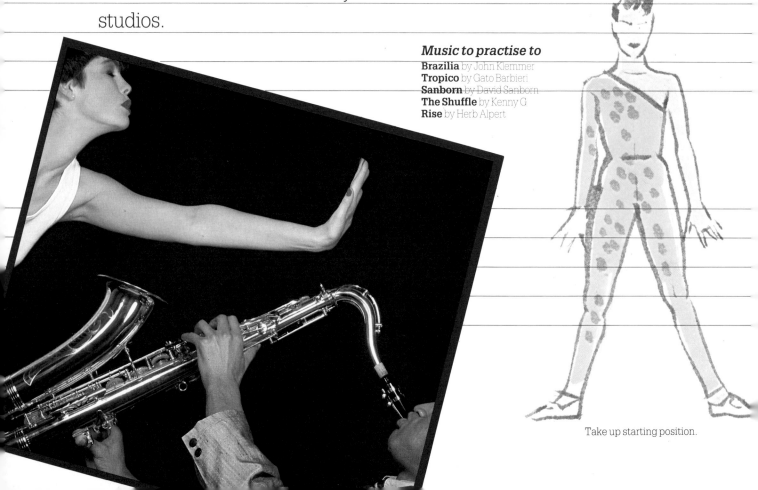

Take up starting position.

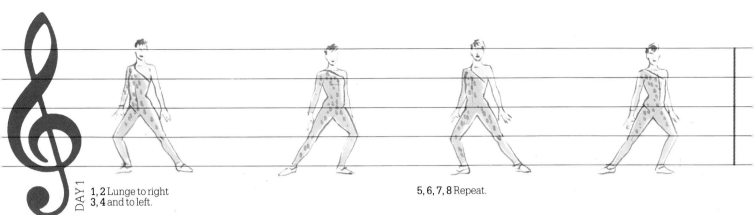

DAY 1

1, 2 Lunge to right
3, 4 and to left.

5, 6, 7, 8 Repeat.

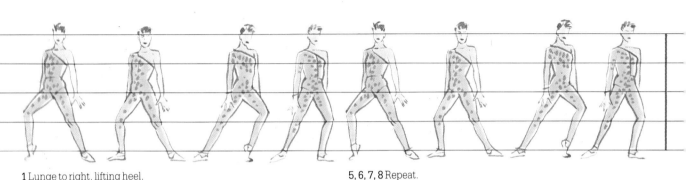

1 Lunge to right, lifting heel,
2 lower heel.
3 Lunge to left, lifting heel
4 lower heel.

5, 6, 7, 8 Repeat.

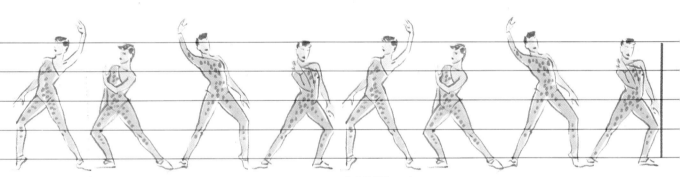

1 Raise left arm and lunge to right, lifting heel
2 and circling arm round in front, lower heel.
3 Raise right arm and lunge to left, lifting heel
4 and circling arm round in front, lower heel.

5, 6, 7, 8 Repeat.

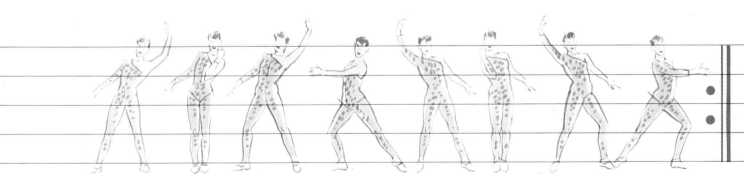

1 Raise left arm and, stepping out with right foot, start circling arm
  above head in lasso action,
2 finishing your circle as you bring in left foot to right foot.
3 Step out to right once more and start to circle upper arm again,
4 this time bringing outstretched arm straight across body, palm facing
  to back, as you bend right knee and lunge forward.

5, 6, 7, 8 Repeat with right arm raised, stepping to left.

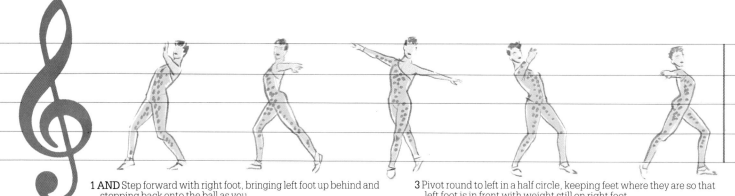

1 AND Step forward with right foot, bringing left foot up behind and stepping back onto the ball as you
2 step forward onto right foot again, bending knee in a lunge. (This movement is easier to do than to read and is called 'step-ball-change'. It has a slight jump at the moment when you transfer the weight from right to left and back to right again, rather like a gallop or a polka step.)

3 Pivot round to left in a half circle, keeping feet where they are so that left foot is in front with weight still on right foot,
AND and step-ball-
4 change with left foot leading, finishing in a lunge with arms to side.

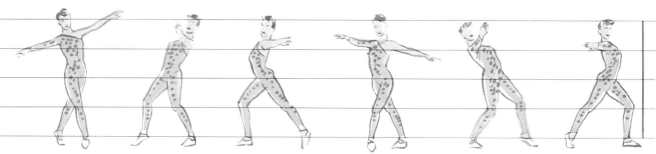

5, 6, 7, 8 Repeat.

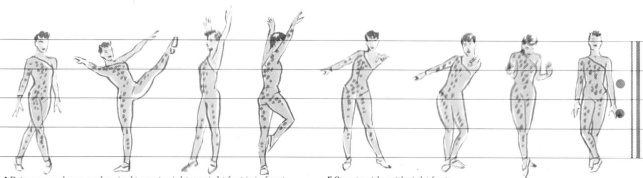

1 Bring arms down and swivel torso to right, so right foot is in front. Take weight onto it
2 and 'Lay-back', kicking leg out to the front, opening arms in a low V.
3 Keeping hands up, return foot to floor, then,
4 transferring weight, bring right toe to left knee and swivel round to right through 360 degrees, lowering arms.

5 Step to side with right foot
6 and swing hip to right, arms in opposition.
7 Contract ribcage (as though punched in stomach), bringing hands up, head down and pointing right foot
8 as you draw it over left foot, bringing hands down, head back.

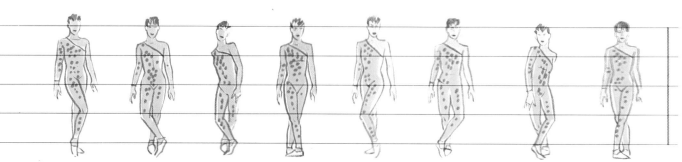

1 Turn right knee in
2 and out again.
3 Plié, pushing left shoulder forwards and across,
4 then return to centre, straightening legs.

5, 6, 7, 8 Repeat, using left knee and right shoulder.

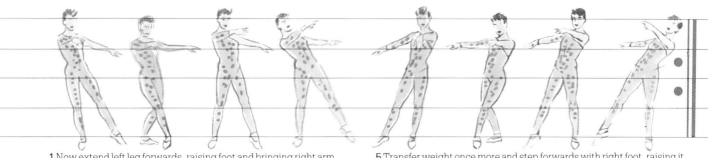

1 Now extend left leg forwards, raising foot and bringing right arm forwards, left arm to side.
2 Bring left foot behind right, plié, then
3 straightening legs, bring right foot to left and transfer your weight onto it,
4 and arch backwards, taking head back and pointing left foot.

5 Transfer weight once more and step forwards with right foot, raising it and changing position of arms, then
6 plié
7 straighten,
8 and arch back.

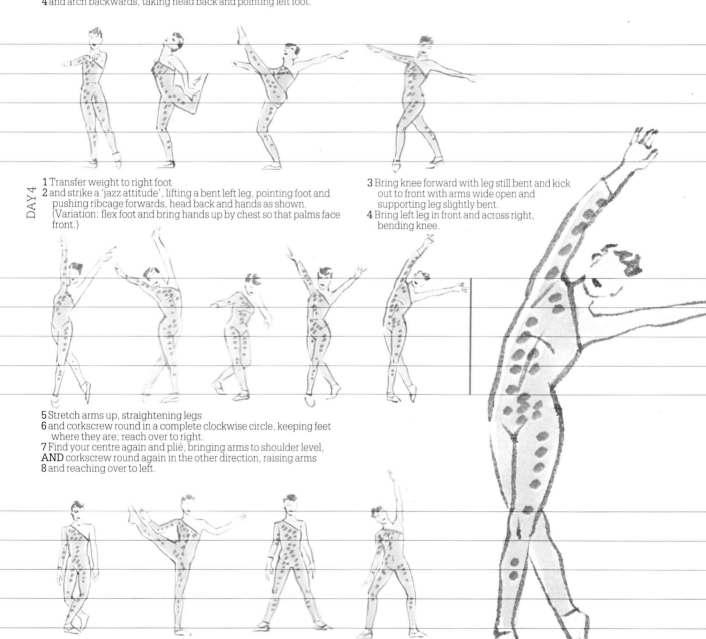

DAY 4

1 Transfer weight to right foot
2 and strike a 'jazz attitude', lifting a bent left leg, pointing foot and pushing ribcage forwards, head back and hands as shown. (Variation: flex foot and bring hands up by chest so that palms face front.)

3 Bring knee forward with leg still bent and kick out to front with arms wide open and supporting leg slightly bent.
4 Bring left leg in front and across right, bending knee.

5 Stretch arms up, straightening legs
6 and corkscrew round in a complete clockwise circle, keeping feet where they are; reach over to right.
7 Find your centre again and plié, bringing arms to shoulder level,
AND corkscrew round again in the other direction, raising arms
8 and reaching over to left.

DAY 5

1 Return to centre, straightening up and bringing arms down; plié,
2 and kick right foot to side with both legs straight and foot pointed.
3 Return foot to floor in second position
4 and raise left arm at the same time as you begin to plié.

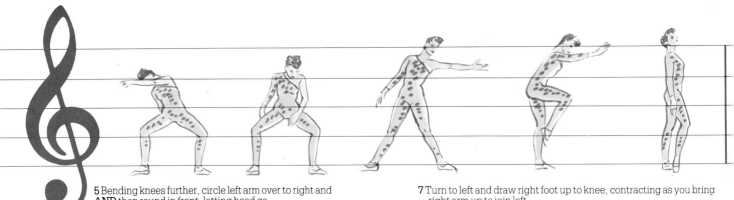

5 Bending knees further, circle left arm over to right and
AND then round in front, letting head go
6 and then straighten it to left.

7 Turn to left and draw right foot up to knee, contracting as you bring right arm up to join left.
8 Lift body, lowering arms and taking head back.

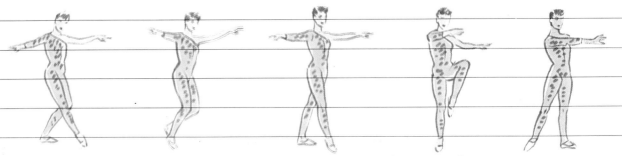

1 Step forwards onto right foot, arms in opposition,
AND and step-ball-change
2 so right foot still leads.

3 Lift left knee, changing arms, then
4 return foot to floor in fourth position.

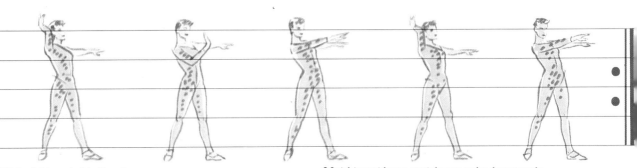

5 Take right arm behind head,
AND then push flexed hand firmly forwards from shoulder,

6 finishing with arm straight out, palm downwards.
7, 8 Repeat.

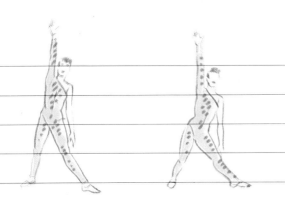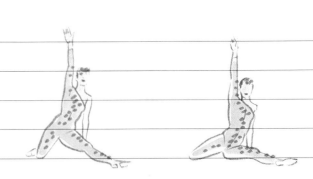

DAY 6 WARM UP WELL BEFORE ATTEMPTING THIS
1, 2 Lower left arm and raise right as you go forwards from hips, sliding front foot forwards and bending back leg.

3 Be prepared to take weight onto left hand as you get lower and let right knee rest on floor,
4 letting body roll to left to sit down, relaxing right knee if necessary.

Using hand to support weight helps prevent pulled muscles, pain in hips . . . but only do this when well warmed up and never go further than feels comfortable.

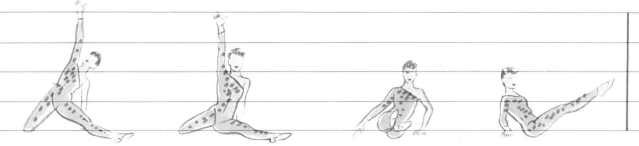

5 Raise right hip, pushing up with left hand and looking up.
6 Return to floor, then

7 take right leg forwards to join left in centre. Lift feet and point them, transferring weight so that it is evenly distributed on sitting bones
8 and swing body and legs round in a half circle to left,

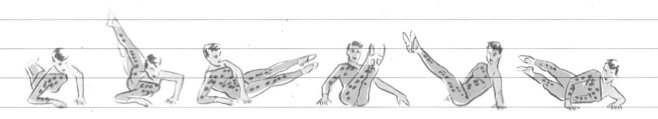

AND 1 bending right knee and letting it rest on floor as you turn onto your front and raise left leg.
2 Push off again and swing round to do the same thing on the other side.

3 so that legs travel round to front, then round to right and behind,
AND 4 bending left knee and letting it rest on floor as you turn onto your front and raise right leg.

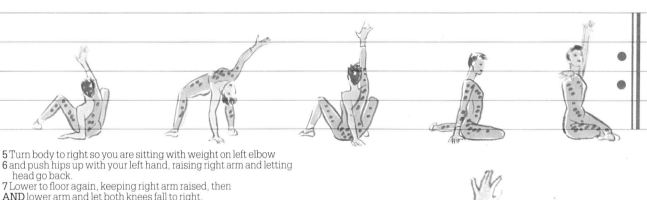

5 Turn body to right so you are sitting with weight on left elbow
6 and push hips up with your left hand, raising right arm and letting head go back.
7 Lower to floor again, keeping right arm raised, then
AND lower arm and let both knees fall to right.
8 Raise left arm up, right arm to side and finish.

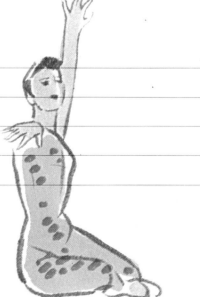

Sports days

Variety is an important part of getting fit. Enjoy sports as well as exercise routines. The key is to choose what you most enjoy, because you will then discover that finding time to exercise ceases to be a problem and becomes a priority – something that you look forward to, enjoy doing and feel good for having done.

The secret is not to expect to continue doing anything for ever – even the most enjoyable activity can pall after a while. Enjoy the challenge of taking up a sport and becoming competent at it, and when you get bored take a break and switch to something new.

On the following pages, you will find training notes and fitness schedules for running, swimming and cycling... basic sports that are reasonably accessible, effective from the fitness point of view and do not require any special expertise, being skills usually learned in childhood.

The schedules are organized in 8 stages: the first is beginner level, the last advanced enough to give heart and lungs substantial aerobic benefits. Start at stage 1 *whatever your level of fitness* and progress stage by stage, graduating only when you feel entirely comfortable with the stage you are on – that means refreshed and energized at the end of a session, not breathless, gasping and nauseous. Aim, ideally, to fit in 3 sessions of your chosen sport a week (or alternate them), but do not try to exercise every day. Rest days are as important as sports days. And remember: these sports days are non-competitive. It's enjoyment that's important, fitness that's the prize.

NB Take your pulse, as directed on page 40, at the start of each new stage as an additional way of monitoring fitness.

RUNNING

RUNNING is simple, easy, accessible, great for mind as well as body, needs little equipment beyond a good pair of training shoes and is one of the most effective ways of getting, and keeping, fit.

RUNNING IS FOR YOU if you are in reasonably good shape before starting.

RUNNING IS NOT FOR YOU if you are very overweight (12.5 kg/2 stone over) as it may place unacceptable strains on heart and joints. Get weight down first, complementing diet with gentle exercise, such as brisk walking or swimming or following the early weeks of the exercise programme. Consult your doctor first if you have problems with heart or high blood pressure, have not exercised for a considerable time or have any doubts about your health.

HOW TO START. Simply get outside for 30 minutes, walking to begin with, then walking/jogging, then jogging and finally running when you feel able. Use the fitness schedule to give you something to aim for, but remember it's not a race: go at your own pace.

Don't run every day; 3 to 4 times a week is quite enough. Rest days will give you a chance to recover energy and help to guard against boredom, keep enthusiasm high.

HOW TO RUN. Sort out your style before you start as postural faults are exaggerated on moving faster. Watch middle-distance (1500-metre) runners on television for an idea of the correct action – legs lifted, upper body still, arms relaxed. Notice, too, that they use the whole of the foot when they run, rolling from heel through to toes. Running on the balls of the feet will not slim thighs or strengthen legs, just tire them unnecessarily. Train on different surfaces – athletic tracks (the best) pavements, parkland, canal towpaths, the beach, up and down hills – and vary the route to help sustain interest.

YOU WILL NEED good quality training shoes. Look for *support* and *cushioning* (at least 2 cm/¾ in on the heel, 1.5 cm/½ in on the sole); *flexibility*, they should bend easily back about a third of the way from the toes; *comfort and fit*, they should feel comfortable right away. Training shoes should never need 'running in'. Also necessary: cotton socks, all-weather tracksuit and jerseys for cold weather, T-shirts, shorts, a good supporting bra and a pedometer (optional).

WARM UP with 10 minutes general stretching. Try yoga sun salutation (116), and general stretches (32, 53, 69). It is particularly important to stretch backs of legs and calves (46, 59 and 39, remembering to hinge forward from hips as you drop down so you feel a stretch along backs of legs).

COOL DOWN by walking the last half-mile home; don't just flake out and stop (see note on page 41). Add a few easy stretches to keep blood flowing to muscles and help guard against stiffness and soreness later.

SUPPLEMENT with mobility exercises for arms (109), shoulders (110) and spine (43, 44, 45); strengtheners for upper body (72, 101) and abdomen (103, 85).

MAKE IT MORE ENJOYABLE: by running with a friend, joining a club, running in the country and on varied surfaces; by taking a pedometer and timing yourself over a given distance or noting down changes in pulse rate, *as instructed on page 40*, and so monitoring progress; by using your imagination – visualize a sail unfurling behind you, a river flowing in the direction you are heading or a breeze blowing – to give you stamina and prevent tiredness taking a hold; by using running time as time off from all the problems and pressures at home – let your attention rest lightly on the moment and feel yourself becoming calmer as your mind becomes quieter.

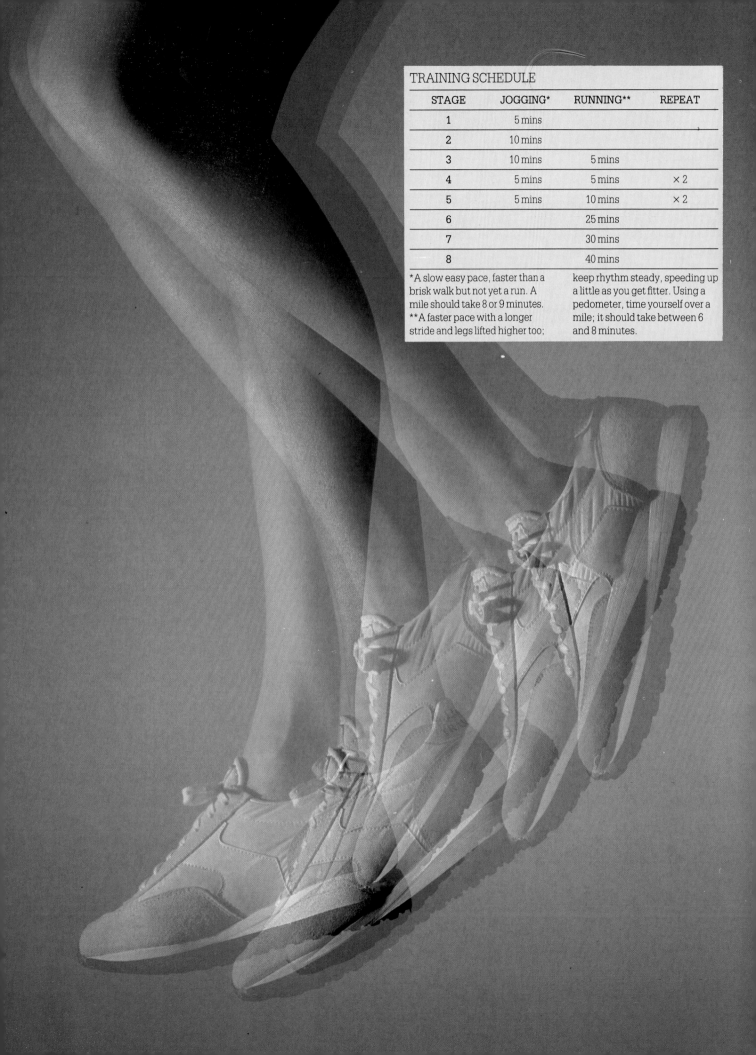

TRAINING SCHEDULE

STAGE	JOGGING*	RUNNING**	REPEAT
1	5 mins		
2	10 mins		
3	10 mins	5 mins	
4	5 mins	5 mins	× 2
5	5 mins	10 mins	× 2
6		25 mins	
7		30 mins	
8		40 mins	

*A slow easy pace, faster than a brisk walk but not yet a run. A mile should take 8 or 9 minutes.
**A faster pace with a longer stride and legs lifted higher too; keep rhythm steady, speeding up a little as you get fitter. Using a pedometer, time yourself over a mile; it should take between 6 and 8 minutes.

CYCLING

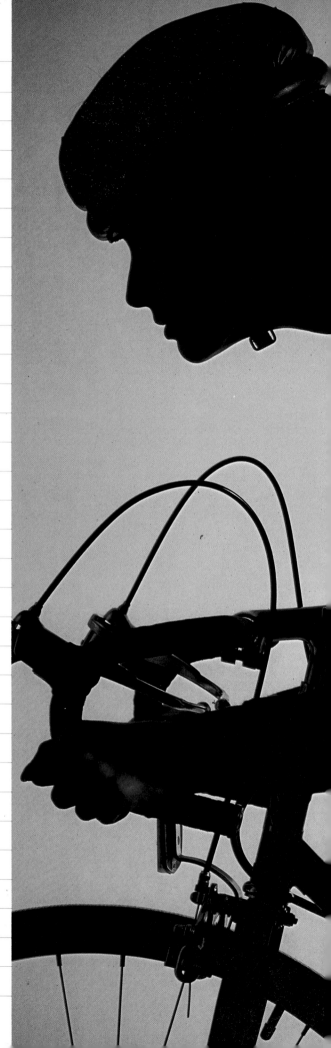

CYCLING is fun and marvellous if you find organized exercise classes a waste of time, because it gets you somewhere as it gets you fit. A car would have to do over 1,000 miles to the gallon to be as economical.

CYCLING IS FOR YOU if you are reasonably fit and have no history of back or knee trouble.

CYCLING IS NOT FOR YOU if you have back trouble or weak knees or consider your leg muscles overdeveloped (take your exercise horizontal instead, *see next page*).

HOW TO START. Gently – in quiet lanes and/or side streets, keeping within a reasonable distance of home. Do not cycle in heavy traffic until confident of cycling ability.

HOW TO CYCLE. With your legs, not your back; crucial to prevent back strain due to muscles shortening and tightening . . . Use your feet as you pedal, rotating ankles and not just pumping legs up and down. Change gears for best training effect: use high ones to pedal fast for heart and health benefits and low ones to increase resistance.

YOU WILL NEED a good bicycle with *height of saddle* adjusted so that you can just balance with toes on the ground while sitting on it, at an *angle* that allows you to sit squarely and not tip forwards. Other necessities: gears, back and front lights, reflector strips, repair kit and instruction manual, pump, lock, bell and maps.

WARM UP with some general stretches, particularly for spine (69, 53) and backs of legs (46, 59). Start off with some slow pedalling to loosen joints, get blood flowing freely.

COOL DOWN with easy pedalling and a few general stretches, particularly backs of legs (59), upper back (4) and chest and shoulders (24) to help prevent stiffness.

SUPPLEMENT WITH mobility exercises for arms (109), shoulders (110) and spine (43, 44, 45); strengtheners for upper body (72, 101) and abdomen (103, 85).

MAKE IT MORE ENJOYABLE by joining a club, cycling with a friend, taking your bicycle on holiday or into the countryside, using maps to explore.

TRAINING SCHEDULE

STAGE	LEISURELY CYCLING	BRISK/UPHILL CYCLING	REPEAT
1	15 mins		
2	10 mins	5 mins	
3	10 mins	5 mins	× 2
4	10 mins	10 mins	× 2
5	15 mins	10 mins	× 2
6	15 mins	15 mins	× 2
7	10 mins	20 mins	× 2
8	10 mins	20 mins	× 3

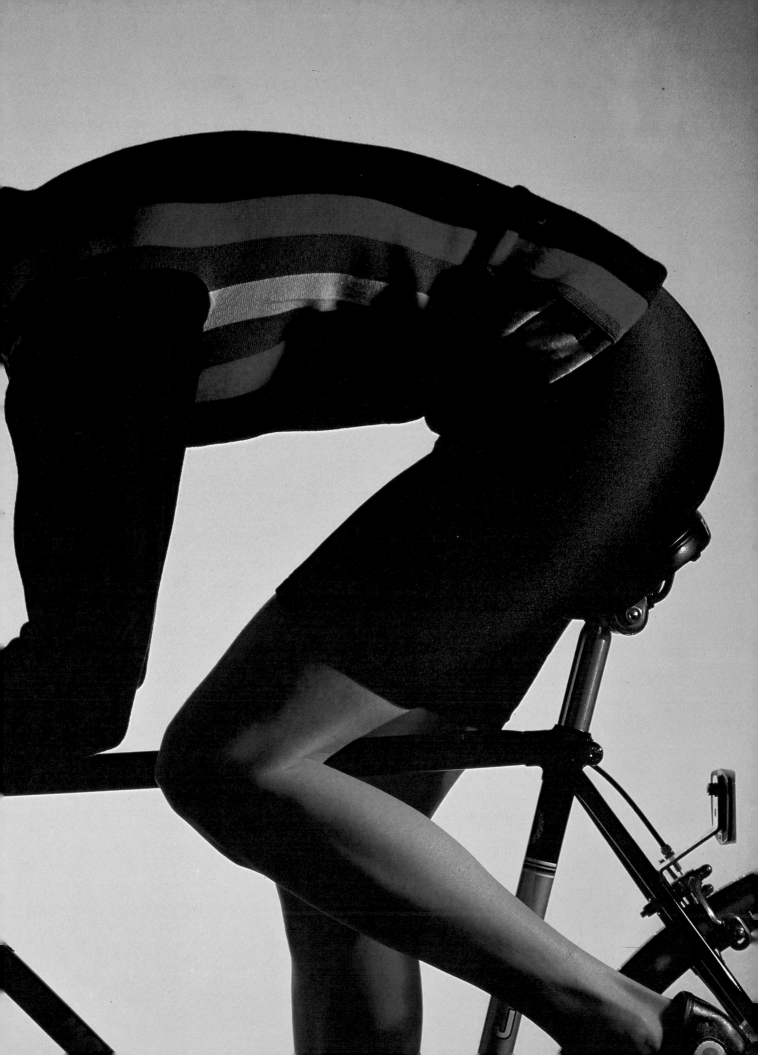

SWIMMING

SWIMMING can be one of the best all-round routes to fitness and relaxing with it. Water removes gravitational pull on bones and joints, so reducing chances of strain or injury, keeps you cool and sweat-free too...

SWIMMING IS FOR YOU if you are very overweight or pregnant, consider your leg muscles overdeveloped, or have joint problems or varicose veins (horizontal position reduces pressure on legs and supporting veins).

SWIMMING IS NOT FOR YOU if you do not have easy access to a pool or have never learned how – though it's never too late to start...

HOW TO START. Purely for pleasure: simply spend about 20 minutes in the pool, and forget about length counting until you feel fit enough to take on the training schedule.

HOW TO SWIM. Lazy breast-stroke or side-stroke up and down the lengths does nothing for heart and lungs, little to tone muscles or promote strength; you must swim fairly vigorously, alternating strokes for best effects. Front crawl gives great aerobic benefits and is a marvellous all-round body conditioner; front butterfly, breast-stroke, back-crawl and back butterfly are all good upper body strengtheners – areas most women do not exercise enough; leg kicks only (back or front holding onto float) streamlines lower body, slimming thighs and firming calves.

YOU WILL NEED a swimming costume cut high at the legs with elasticated straps, a swimcap to protect hair from chlorine or salt, earplugs or goggles if susceptible to ear or eye infections, a float to hold on to for leg-kick-only lengths, towel, hairdrier and warm clothes.

WARM UP with a few minutes general stretching and one or two easy lengths to help stretch muscles and prepare them for more vigorous work.

COOL DOWN with one or two easy lengths and some dry-land stretching.

SUPPLEMENT with some twists for the spine (43, 44, 45); strengtheners for abdomen (103, 85).

TRAINING SCHEDULE

STAGE	SWIMMING	LEG-KICK ONLY	'RESTING' STROKE*	REPEAT
1	2 mins	1 min	2 mins	× 3
2	4 mins	1 min	2 mins	× 3
3	3 mins	1 min	2 mins	× 4
4	4 mins	1 min	2 mins	× 4
5	4 mins	2 mins	2 mins	× 4
6	4 mins	1 min	1 min	× 6
7	5 mins	1 min	1 min	× 6
8	4 mins	1 min	1 min	× 8

Alternate a length of crawl with a length of breastroke; a length of crawl with a length of backstroke, and so on; incorporate butterfly, too, if you can do it.

*A long easy stroke on back or front.

102

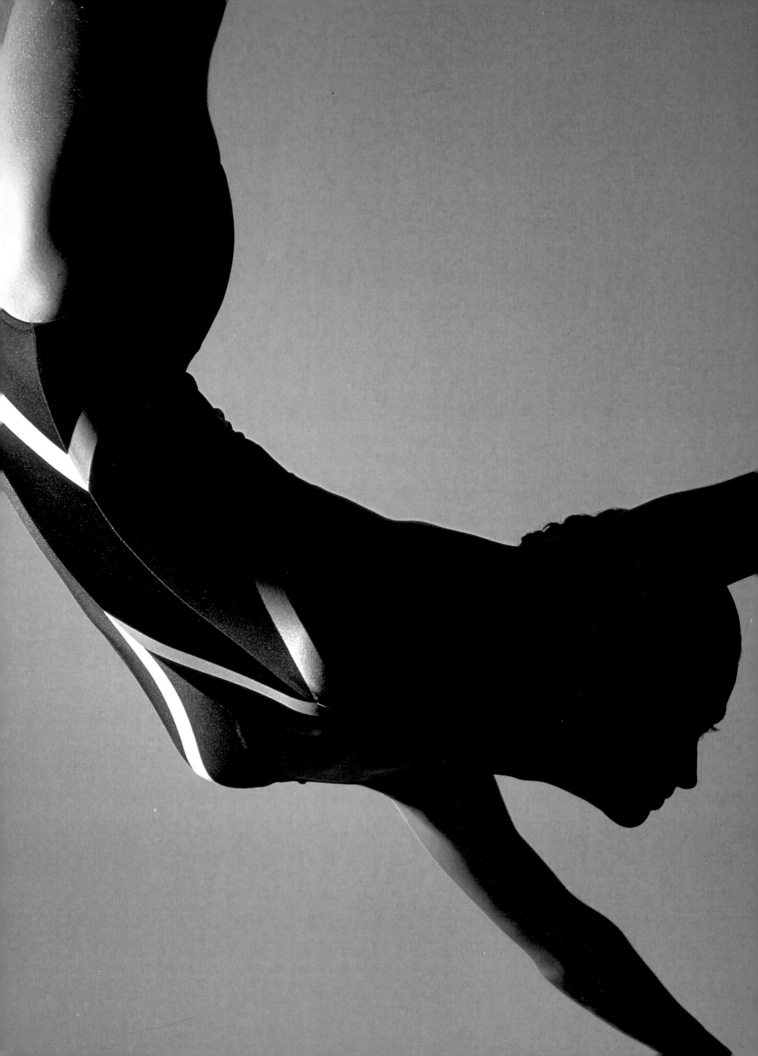

Pre-ski programme

The best guarantee of enjoyment on a skiing holiday is a strong, fit body because skiing makes great demands on muscles and joints. Here is a specially devised pre-ski programme to get you into top physical condition before leaving for the slopes. Give yourself at least 3 weeks to get fit and include an aerobic activity, such as jogging or skipping, to help build up stamina.

WARM UP well first to ease stiffness, lengthen muscles and loosen joints. Suggested sequence: 116, 32, 53, 69, 46 and 39.

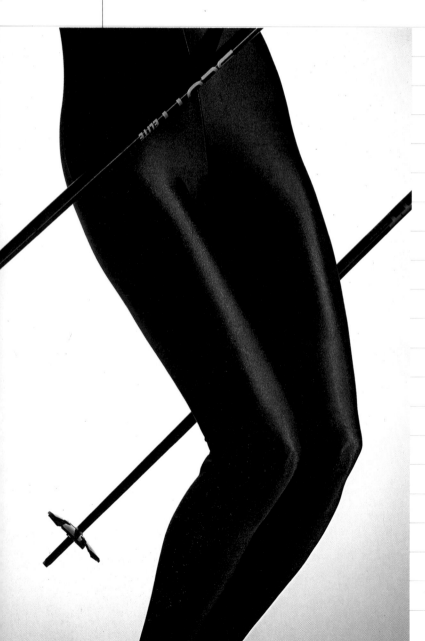

ARMS AND SHOULDERS
Take arms up to shoulder level and make loose fists. Circle them backwards several times, breathing well. Add 0.5 kg/1 lb weights to make this mobility exercise a strengthener too.

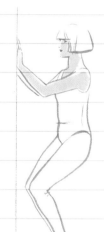

THIGHS *Stand with back to wall and gradually bend knees until sitting with thighs parallel to the floor. Stay there until muscles tire, gradually building up holding time to 1½ minutes.*

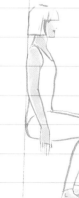

THIGHS *Stand with hands on wall, as shown, and bend knees. Bounce lightly up and down and continue until muscles tire.*

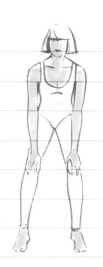
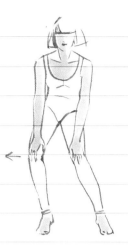
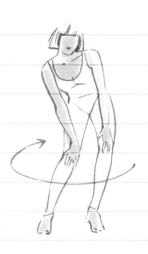

HIPS, KNEES AND ANKLES

Stand with knees slightly bent and feet hip-width apart. Place hands on knees, as shown, and sway from side to side in a good rhythm transferring your weight smoothly. Progress to making circles with your knees in both directions, clockwise and anti-clockwise, and finally try making figures-of-eight.

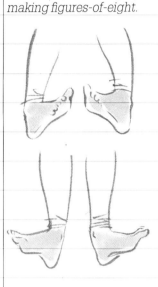

ANKLES
Sit with knees together and heels apart. Bring big toes, together, trying to lift them up as much as possible. Then brush outwards along floor again, pulling little toes upwards and pressing big toes down. Repeat until ankles and calves tire.
Strong, mobile ankles are important for maintaining balance, absorbing impact.

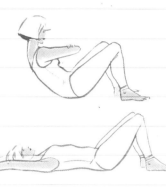

ABDOMEN
Sit with legs bent and feet hip-width apart. Breathe out as you bring chin towards chest, rounding back and lowering yourself backwards, pulling forwards with elbows at same time. Hold at point where you feel abdominal muscles tightening to prevent you falling backwards. Repeat several times.
Now lie down on the floor and curl up, breathing out and bringing arms in front. Start by holding for 2 seconds and try to build to slow count of 5, but do not attempt to curl up any further than shown. Repeat several times. Progress to hands by your sides, arms folded in front and, finally, fingers interlocked behind head. Repeat exercise to either side to work diagonal abdominal muscles, pulling well across body with top arm each time.

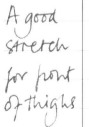

FRONT OF BODY
Sitting on heels, breathe in. As you breathe out, push buttocks upwards. Walk hands back along floor so spine stays lengthened as you arch up, letting head drop gently back. Hold for a few moments, then release.

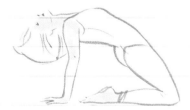

FALLING
Falling is inevitable when skiing. Help overcome your fear of it by practising falling onto a soft sprung surface, letting your body drop and loosen into the movement rather than tensing and resisting it.

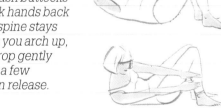

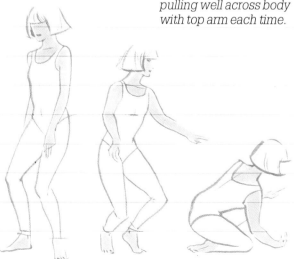

Exercising
for childbirth

If keeping yourself fit with the exercises in this book is part of your normal routine, you will find very little change is necessary when you become pregnant. The same is true after the birth, when you should just work gradually from the first week of the programme until you attain your normal level of fitness. There are nevertheless some exercises which you will find particularly helpful and these are set out here.

Best to avoid during pregnancy: sports which involve running or jumping unless already used to them; lying on your front as soon as this becomes uncomfortable; lying on your back if this becomes uncomfortable or makes you feel breathless in late pregnancy; back bends if your back is giving you trouble.

Once used to this, try it away from wall, kneeling on all-fours, lying on back with knees bent (not in late pregnancy if uncomfortable), on your side and any other way you can think of.

BEFORE

PELVIC TILT

This important movement lengthens muscles of lower back and helps keep abdominal muscles strong enough to take weight of growing baby. Start against a wall so you cannot cheat by moving top half as well. Feet should be slightly apart and away from wall and *knees slightly bent. Feel back of head, shoulder blades and spine resting against wall and breathe in. As you breathe out, press back of waist into wall so that bottom moves away from it a little. This is a very small movement. Repeat several times slowly with correct breathing.*

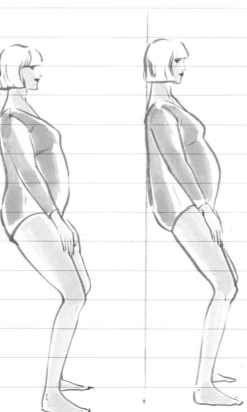

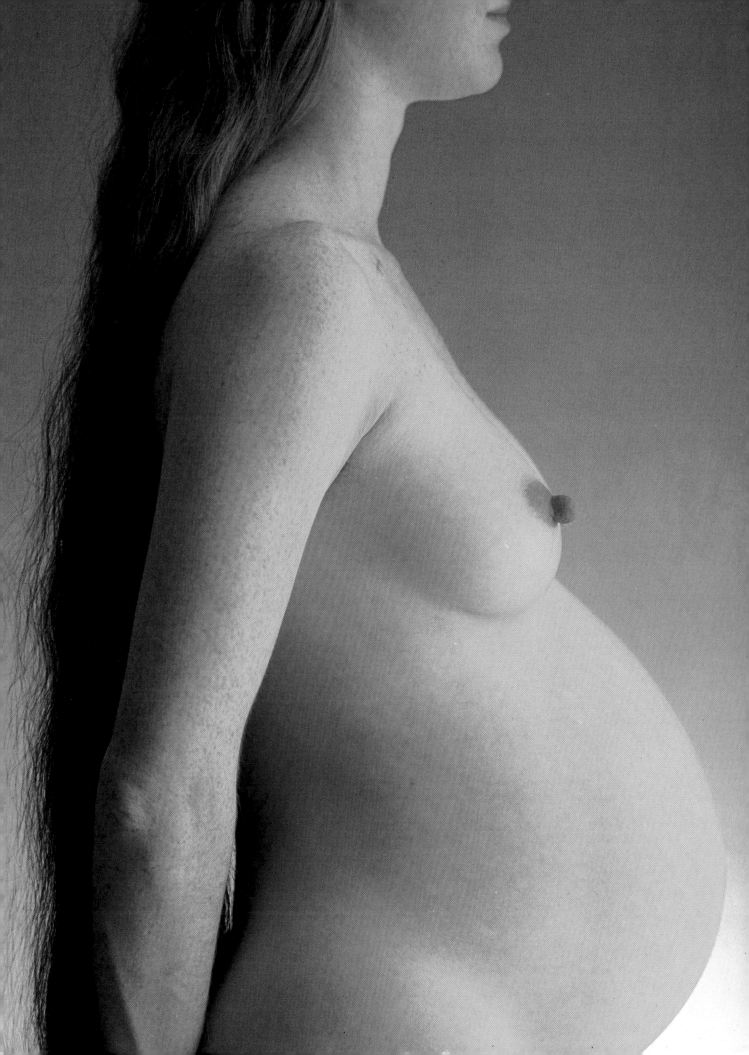

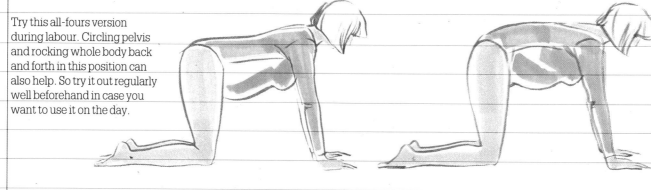

Try this all-fours version during labour. Circling pelvis and rocking whole body back and forth in this position can also help. So try it out regularly well beforehand in case you want to use it on the day.

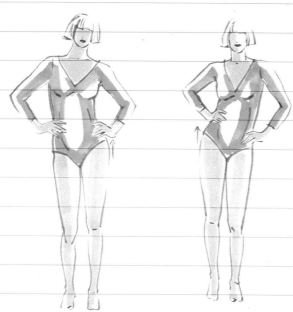

Although it is important to be fit and strong for birth, you should not overstrain yourself during pregnancy (or, indeed, at any time) and that includes forcing yourself to take exercise when you don't feel like it. Listen to your body, and if you feel like taking a great deal of rest, take it – particularly in the first months when you may find you are much more tired than usual. If you stay in tune with your needs and those of your baby, you will find that the day will come when you feel like doing some gentle movements to keep your body strong and supple, ready for the remarkable physical feat of giving birth.

SIDEWAYS PELVIC TILT

Standing with feet apart, lift left hip towards left ribs and then right hip towards right ribs. Repeat several times, transferring smoothly from side to side with a good rhythm, and then try it with knees bent.

Mobility of the pelvis is essential for comfort during pregnancy and is also very important during labour, especially if you wish to have an active birth when you will be using your body to help you and the baby in every way you can.

PELVIC ROTATIONS *Try this kneeling down at first so that you can practise circling pelvis slowly all the way round, clockwise and anti-clockwise, without swaying from thighs. Then enjoy it standing, with knees slightly bent.*

Rocking movements are very soothing for you and your baby and you may find them useful in labour

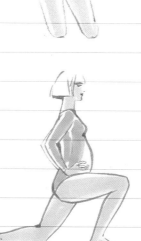

PELVIC ROCKING *Try rocking pelvis to and fro in a half-kneeling position, allowing thighs to rock too.*

POSTURE CHECK

Starting from your pelvis, check that you are centred and not tipping lower part of pelvis back, shortening and arching your back (this is a very common fault in pregnancy as the bulge grows in front). Check, too, that you are not throwing pelvis too far forwards into pelvic tilt position (this is rarer). Now ask yourself these questions: Is weight evenly distributed between heels and balls of feet with arches well lifted in centre? Are knees at ease and neither pushed too far back nor bent? Is spine lengthened right up to base of skull, so that you feel as though you are being pulled upwards from centre of crown of head? Are shoulders sloping down as far away from ears as possible? Is head balanced easily on neck with chin at about a right angle to throat? Is lower jaw free or is it pressed upwards so that teeth are clenched (practise yawning if it is)? Are arms hanging freely by sides and hands unclenched?

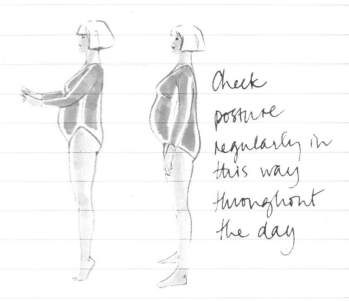

Check posture regularly in this way throughout the day

A supple lengthened spine is especially important during pregnancy because it helps prevent the aches and pains that poor posture can cause as you get heavier, particularly back-ache. It will also help you to make maximum room both for the baby and for your breathing. The ribs are the correct breathing apparatus and, if your spine is lengthened, the whole of your ribcage, which goes nearly down to your waist at the back, will be free to work properly.

...ur partner ...ld apply ...ttle ...ssure as ...n breathe

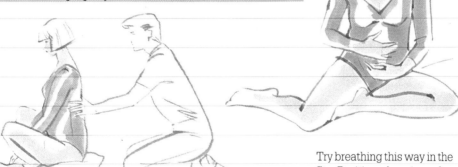

Exercising becomes much less of an effort if you make it a part of your daily life. The Star Positions given here can be used whenever you feel like it – not just reserved for a special exercise 'time'. They are excellent preparation for an active birth as they prepare the legs and hips, strengthen and lengthen the back and give you a good chance to practise your breathing. Think of the stretches as active relaxation exercises that will benefit you both while you are pregnant and once labour begins. Use your breathing to help you remain calm throughout . . .

BREATHING

Sit in any comfortable position where spine is lengthened and ribs are free and concentrate on taking each breath down to the baby and then letting each breath out completely. Think about your baby as you do this. Stroking and circular movements with palms of hands over the bump will be comforting for you both too. Breathe down to the baby at back of body as well, getting a friend to check that you are using whole of ribcage at back by placing hands just above your waist at the back, as shown, and allowing hands to rise and fall with your breathing, so that you can really feel expansion of lower ribs in middle of back.

Try breathing this way in the Star Positions, keeping calm and relaxed as you breathe through the stretch.

STAR POSITIONS

FROG POSITION ★

Kneel on a mat or soft surface with toes together and knees apart – eventually aiming to get bottom to touch floor. Now walk hands forwards, with palms on floor, so that you gradually lower body. But try to lengthen out spine completely, placing forehead on a cushion as shown or stretching arms in front if you prefer. Stay there for at least a minute if you can (2 when you get used to it), breathing well and emphasizing out-breath so you stay relaxed.

Don't worry if toes come apart a little

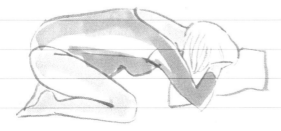

You will probably feel an intense stretch in groin area, so use it to practise labour breathing and relaxation.

COBBLER POSE ★

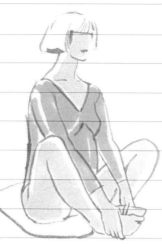

Sit on a cushion or two with knees bent and soles of feet together as close to you as possible. Holding onto feet or ankles, lengthen back, lifting ribs away from hips. At the same time, drop shoulders down away from ears. Hold position, breathing well. Flop, letting back round, and then try again, gradually working towards holding position for up to 2 minutes. Then take hands behind you, lean on them and do a pelvic tilt gently dropping thighs towards floor several times when you feel you can take the stretch.

It is a good idea to do this with a partner sitting opposite as shown, so that you get a really good stretch. Breathe and release into it, practising labour breathing and paying full attention to your body.

If you feel a very strong stretch in some of these positions, don't tighten up to protect yourself from it as you may want to do, but breathe through it instead, as if it were a labour contraction, concentrating particularly on the out-breaths. Build up until you can hold the stretch for a full minute. Complete attention is necessary so that you can distinguish between an intense stretch (which will nearly always subside as you accept it and breathe through it, staying relaxed and calm) and acute pain. If you feel acute pain, come out of the position immediately and tell your doctor about it.

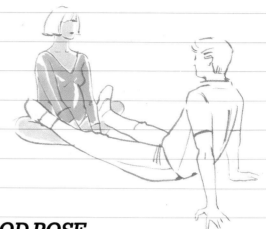

Don't worry if you feel very stiff to begin with. As your pregnancy progresses, a hormone will be released which will soften the ligaments and loosen your joints in order to increase the size of the pelvis and so accommodate the growing baby. The later months of pregnancy are therefore an excellent time to work on increasing general mobility. You may find you become so supple that you can put yourself into positions never achieved before.

ROD POSE (WITH FORWARD BEND) ★

Still sitting on cushions, stretch legs out in front with knees facing ceiling, insides of feet touching. Place a belt or towel around balls of feet and, gently pulling against it, slowly lengthen up back to vertical, or as near as possible. Hold breathing well and, when you feel you can take more stretch, go forwards from the hips keeping back straight (as exercise 39 in Exercise Programme). Eventually you should be able to rest chest on thighs, head on calves or supported on a towel folded onto calves.

This also helps to relieve cramp in calves

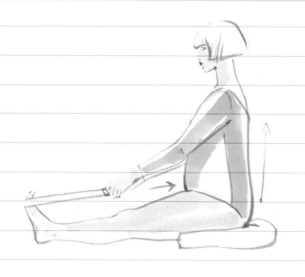

'V' POSITION ★

Sitting with legs apart, press against inside thighs to lift spine up to vertical. Hold as you feel stretch, remembering to think of it like a contraction and breathing through it, staying calm and relaxed.

Do these exercises with back against a wall if they prove too much at first. Eventually your back should be vertical. Check progress from time to time by doing exercise sideways on to a mirror.

Prepare yourself physically and psychologically for labour by gradually increasing your holding time on the strong stretches given here. Once you can hold them for 2 minutes or more, breathing well, you can be confident in your ability to remain calm and relaxed on the day, for your labour contractions will never last longer than 1¾ minutes. If you find the stretches become less intense as you get more supple, take the positions further until the intensity increases again...

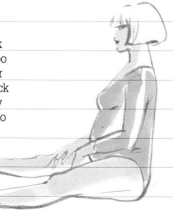

SQUATTING ★

This traditional birthing position gives lower back an excellent stretch and also stretches groin area and thighs, so it is very useful both during pregnancy and in preparation for the birth itself. Try it holding onto a chair or other support at first or leaning back against a wall and sliding down. It does not matter if heels don't touch floor, but if they do, it will give calves a useful stretch.

Try pelvic floor exercise in this position. Control is good if you can squeeze and lift pelvic floor with legs so wide apart.

DAILY MAINTENANCE

PELVIC FLOOR
To locate your pelvic floor muscles, test them out while you are passing water (not on an extremely full bladder though, such as first thing in the morning) by stopping flow of urine mid-stream. You should be able to stop it completely with no drips. If you can't, pelvic floor muscles need working on. Lift them up a little (as though stopping urine flow mid-stream), then a little more, more

again, and finally lift and squeeze upwards as much as you can. Hold for a slow count of 5 and then lower in 3 stages as before. Don't worry if you can't get all stages up or down at first – you will become more precise with practice. Try to do this at least 5 times a day. Lift and squeeze pelvic floor in one quick movement too and repeat several times daily. When you are familiar with exercise, try combining it with pelvic tilt. Use it during love-making too.

The sling of muscle at the bottom of pelvis has a big weight-bearing job to do as pregnancy progresses and is stretched to the limit during childbirth itself.

LEG SWINGS
These will get circulation moving in hips and legs. Try them forwards and back and across and out away from body, holding lightly onto the back of a chair for support.

The first and most essential ost·natal exercise o get used to it now

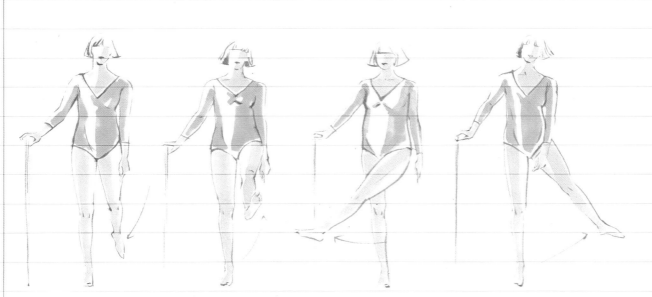

111

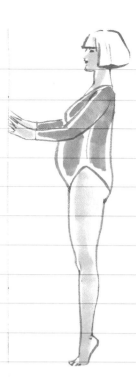

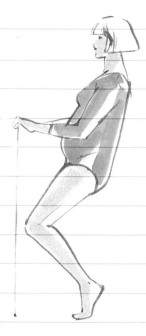

CALF FIRMER

This will also get circulation going. Standing with feet together and fingertips on a support, raise up onto balls of feet, as shown, lower heels half-way to floor and then push up again. Repeat energetically several times until calves begin to tire. Shake legs well.

FRONT OF THIGH FIRMER

Standing as left, lift up onto balls of feet. Do a pelvic tilt and bend knees, let them separate. Do 4 small further bends so front of thighs are working strongly, then straighten legs fully still up on toes. Repeat several times till front of thighs tire. Give legs a good shake-out.

Walks in the fresh air are marvellous exercise, as is swimming. If you are fit and have been doing yoga for some time, it would be an excellent idea to continue with your classes, avoiding positions such as lying on your tummy or advanced twists when these become uncomfortable. Once you have adjusted your shoulder stand to take your new-found weight, you may find being upside-down a great relief.

SIDE STRETCH

Sitting cross-legged, breathe in and stretch one arm up over head. Reach over to opposite side, enjoying stretch and breathing out. Breathe in as you return to centre and then change arms and stretch to other side. Repeat several times.

Makes a useful recovery exercise between strong stretches

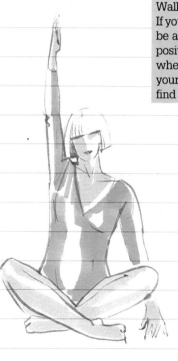

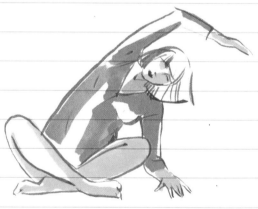

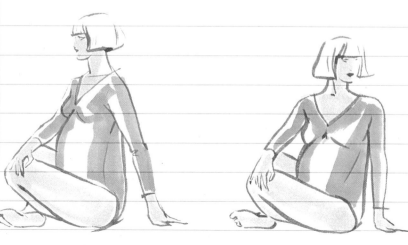

TWIST *Sitting cross-legged, place one hand on opposite knee and press the other into floor behind you to help lift spine as you take a good breath in. As you breathe out, twist gently round towards arm at back and look round gently too. Think of spiralling round on a well-lifted spine as you do this. Hold for a few moments, breathing normally, then repeat to other side.*

COMPLETE RELAXATION

First make sure you are warm enough, covering yourself with a blanket if necessary, and then make yourself comfortable. The position shown here is often the most comfortable in late pregnancy, so try it out and see if you like it (the cushion under the knee is useful for added comfort as is another cushion under tummy). Or try lying on back (providing this is still comfortable) with legs raised on a support about 45 cm (18 ins) above heart; or with a cushion or two under thighs to ease lower back. Whichever position you choose, start by doing a few pelvic tilts to make sure spine is lengthened. Pull shoulders down away from ears. Feel the tension release in the neck and shoulders as you do this. Spread arms a little away from body, quieten your mind by focusing on the rhythm of your breathing and take one or two deep breaths down to the baby. Then let breathing fall into its own rhythm, which will become lighter as you relax more deeply. Check through body to see if anything is tight. Are you holding onto a frown or clenching jaws? Are you tensing hands, tummy muscles, thighs, calves, toes? Let go and feel yourself easing further into floor with each out-breath. Allow yourself to be completely supported. When you have finished, take a few deep breaths, raise arms above head and have a good stretch – then get up SLOWLY. First bend knees, then roll onto side if you are lying on your back.

Find out as much as you can through books and ante-natal classes, and by asking questions at your hospital before the birth so that you are aware of all the choices open to you. This may include choosing what type of pain relief you want, if any; deciding whether you would like to give birth in the conventional legs-up position or would like to try something more active, such as squatting; and letting your doctor or midwife know how you, your partner and your baby would like to be treated immediately after the birth.

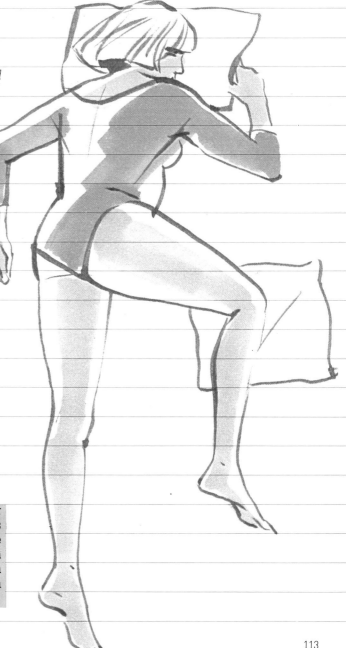

Do a little pelvic tilt to prevent back arching when you raise arms above head into stretch at the end.

Try this routine standing and sitting as well as lying and use it several times a day

Set aside at least 20 minutes at some point of the day for Complete Relaxation and try to keep the rest of your day as calm and unrushed as possible. On very busy days, use the relaxation technique to centre you again and top you up with the calmness and energy you need to carry on. Use it, too, as a time to communicate with your growing baby so that you can begin to get to know each other.

AFTER THE BIRTH

The best post-natal tummy exercise is laughter. Add some serious work with the pelvic floor muscles and abdomen and a few movements to keep the circulation going in the legs if you are not yet up and around much and you will have everything you need for the first few days after the birth. After about a week – or as soon as you feel ready, start on the post-natal programme given here. This 5-minute routine should be carried out twice daily and continued for 12 weeks. Once you have had a 3-month check-up, and provided that your doctor agrees you are in good shape, you should be ready to return to the first week of the general programme.

If you have had a Caesarian birth, work your feet and ankles (see feet exercises, opposite) and start lifting and squeezing the pelvic floor muscles as soon as you can. Very soon, you will be able to begin a very gentle tummy exercise – simply pull your tummy in on an out-breath – and add the pelvic tilts as soon as you can. Once you are up and around, you will probably be ready to start the post-natal programme, but check with your doctor first.

If you have had stitches, you may be worried about exercising the pelvic floor. In fact, these exercises will help healing, and cannot possibly harm the stitches.

IMMEDIATELY AFTERWARDS

PELVIC FLOOR LIFTS
The first and most essential post-natal exercise. Do 4 slow and a few quick lifts at least 4 times and continue for at least 3 months, when you can try the test at the end of this section.

The pelvic floor muscles are stretched to the limit during childbirth, so working them is essential if they are to be restored to full strength. Start as soon as possible after the delivery, lifting and squeezing the pelvic floor several times daily and doing a few quick squeezes too. You will now be thankful you practised these in pregnancy for although you may feel practically no sensation at first, you will at least know what to aim for! Keep practising your pelvic floor lifts regularly so that by the time your baby is 3 months old you can lift your pelvic floor up 4 levels and down 3 without any trouble at all.

PELVIC TILTS

Lie on bed with shoulders down away from ears and spine in a nice straight line, knees bent and feet flat on bed. Place hands on tummy to help you feel what you are doing. Breathe in. As you breathe out, press back of waist firmly into mattress, contracting tummy muscles at the same time. Hold for a few seconds and then breathe in and release. Repeat several times and combine with pelvic floor lifts as soon as you get the idea.

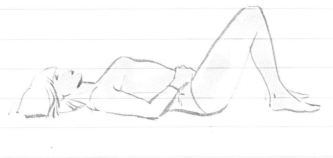

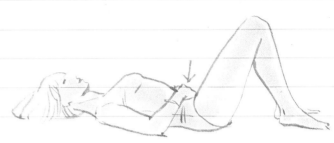

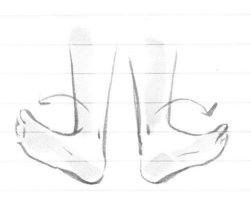

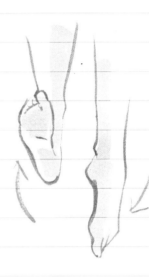

FEET EXERCISES

Keep circulation going with feet rotations, clockwise and anti-clockwise, and then try pedalling – first one foot downwards as the other comes up and then both down and up together. Repeat several times throughout the day.

POST-NATAL PROGRAMME

Start a week after the birth or as your physiotherapist advises.

PELVIC FLOOR LIFTS
As previous page.

PELVIC TILTS FOR TIGHTENING TUMMY
As above. Whenever you think of it plus 4 times lying on your back before your afternoon rest and again at night.

Great for tightening tummy.
Try squeezing buttocks together

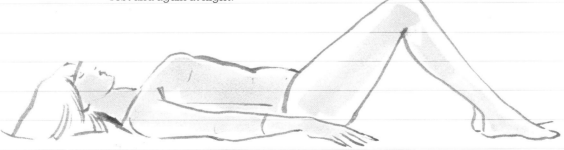

115

STRAIGHT CURL-UPS

Lie on bed with arms at sides, legs bent and feet flat. Breathe in. As you breathe out, lift head and shoulders and pull forwards with hands. (At first, you may only be able to lift head, but persevere.) Breathe in and return to bed. Build up until you can repeat slowly 4 times and then progress by holding curl-up for longer.

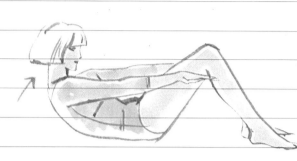

If you feel yourself straining front of neck when you lift head and shoulders, return head to the bed and roll it from side to side a few times or place a cushion or two under head before starting.

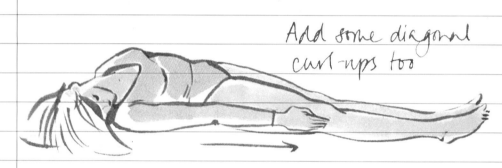

Add some diagonal curl-ups too

CURL-UPS WITH SIDE BENDS

Lie as before, but with arms at sides and hands touching thighs. Breathe in. As you breathe out, lift head and slide right hand down towards outside right knee as far as you can. Then change to left side. Try to repeat twice each side and then rest. Build up to 4 slow repetitions each side.

DIAGONAL CURL-UPS

Lie as before, but with arms about 30 cm (12 ins) away from body. Breathe in. As you breathe out, lift head and take left hand across body to touch right. Lower to bed again and repeat to other side. Try it 4 times slowly on alternating sides.

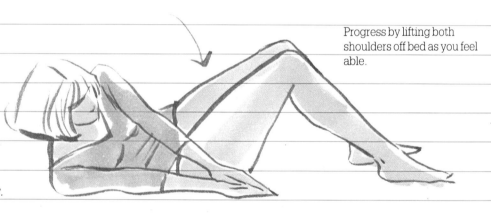

Progress by lifting both shoulders off bed as you feel able.

LEG SLIDES

Lie in a long straight line and slowly bend up one leg and then stretch it out again with foot moving along bed. Repeat with other leg. KEEP BACK PRESSED FIRMLY INTO BED THROUGHOUT. Repeat several times slowly, and then more quickly, allowing one leg to come up as the other goes down in a pedalling action.

Increase the number of repetitions on each exercise as the days go by. But don't tire yourself. It is better to do a few several times a day than a large amount all at once.

Place hands under either side of waist to check you are keeping back down.

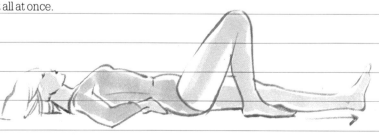

LEG ROLLS Lying
with arms out sideways,
legs bent and feet flat, roll
legs to one side as far as
feels reasonably
comfortable and then to
the other. Press back firmly
into bed each time you
pass through central
position and repeat several
times slowly, and then
more quickly as you feel
able.

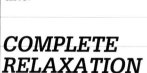

COMPLETE RELAXATION
Practise 20 minutes daily –
or, at worst, 5 minutes 4
times a day.

AFTER 3 MONTHS

TEST PELVIC FLOOR Standing
with feet apart, leap up and
down in the air several
times coughing as you do
so. You should be able to
do this without the
slightest hint of a leak. If all
is not in order, report to
your doctor.

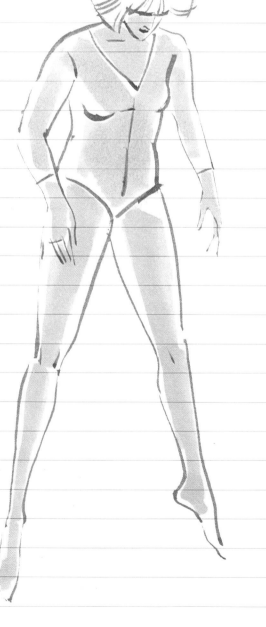

Therapeutics

Exercise should ultimately solve problems by making you fitter and healthier, but it often does so by bringing problems to light first. When you start to exercise, you will find that you become more aware of your body, of both its possibilities *and* its limitations. As your range of movement increases, you may become conscious of tensions which you had not noticed before but which were undoubtedly there all along – stiffness in the lower spine, a taut muscle at the side of the neck, less mobility in one hip than the other ... This inner awareness is the first step to self-help. You must know what is amiss before you can hope to find ways of dealing with it.

The target, then, is to know yourself better than anyone else knows you – and that includes the 'specialists' to whom you might entrust your health. When you take responsibility for your body, you start to feel confident in your own abilities – not least the ability to look after yourself and to find effective ways of making yourself feel better. Massage and movement, you will discover, are two of the best.

This section is divided into three parts. The first part uses massage and movement sequences, the latter largely Feldenkrais-inspired, to help overcome stiffness and loss of mobility in 'problem' areas. Everyone will benefit from them, achieving more freedom and fluidity of movement and so gaining more from their exercising. The second part deals with problems that might occur as a direct result of exercise, such as leg cramps, and gives some practical self-help suggestions. The last part uses movement and massage techniques to help relieve common problems and disorders – much better than reaching for drugs... And, remember, exercise is not only therapeutic but also one of the best ways of safeguarding the good health that you have.

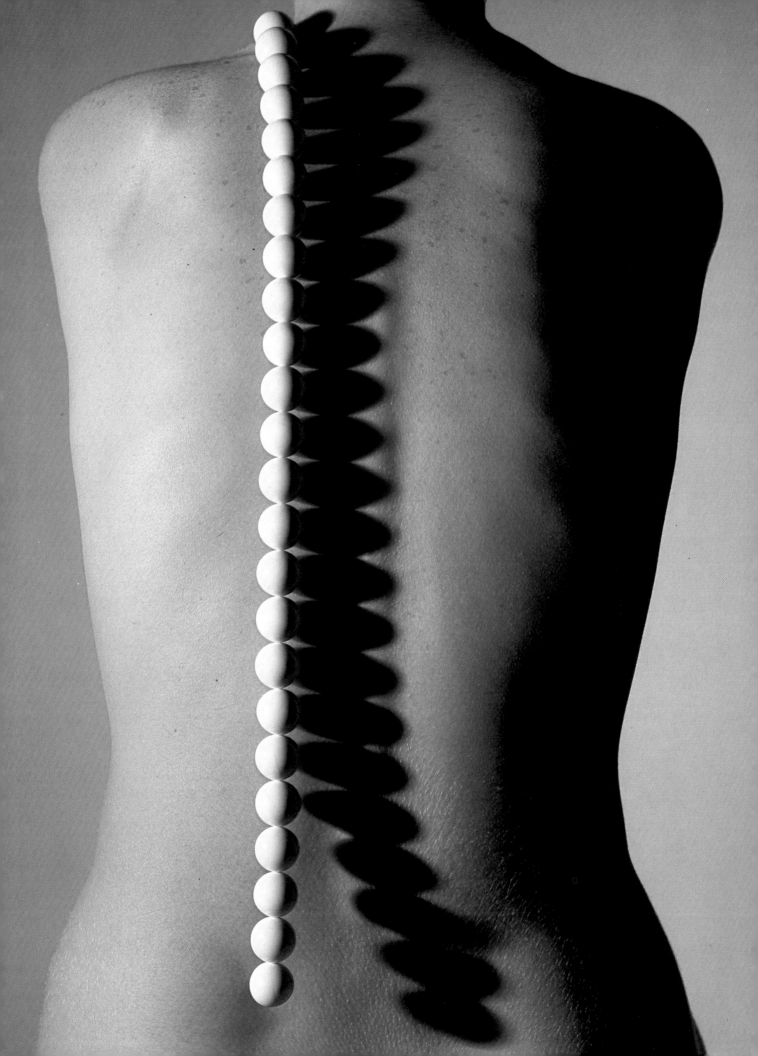

PART 1
NECK AND SHOULDERS

I. Lie on floor and place hand on forehead. Letting hand lead forehead, turn head to right, back to centre and then slowly over to left. Repeat several times, noting how far head moves and quality of movement. Keeping hand on forehead, let head lead hand as you turn it from side to side several times. Take hand away and repeat several times, slowly and easily, breathing well. Rest.

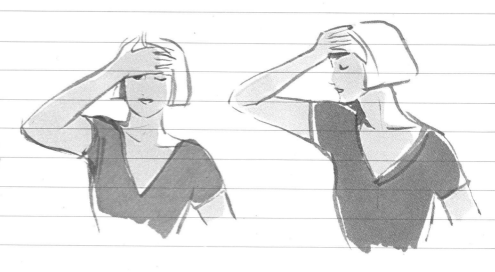

Helps ease tension at back of neck and throat

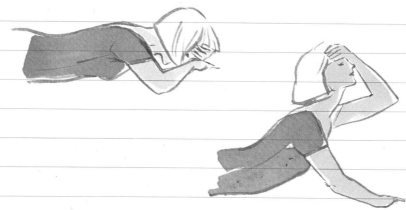

II. Roll onto front. Place one hand on top of the other, the first palm down, the second palm up with forehead resting on it. Let this hand lightly lift head up and back so chest and upper back come off floor. Do not force movement, just go as far as is comfortable, noting quality and extent of movement. Repeat several times, then change hands. Rest a moment.

III. Lie with both hands above forehead, as shown, right cheek on floor. Lift head, keeping right cheek parallel to floor, and move back of head towards right elbow. Pass through centre and move forehead towards left elbow. Rest cheek lightly on floor again and check for signs of tension. Are your fists clenched? Your jaws tight? Your eyes staring? Are you frowning? Release these tensions and repeat movement several times, remaining aware of your breathing. Then turn head, so left cheek is resting on floor, and repeat several times. Rest a moment.

A NOTE ABOUT PAIN. Pain is the body's most basic warning that all is not well. Never ignore it, hoping that it will go away, because it is *always* there for a reason. It might be the way you are doing the exercises and using, or misusing, your body or it might be something much more fundamental. The sooner you find out what is causing it and why, enlisting the help of your doctor if necessary, the closer you will be to taking that pain away permanently.

Loosens shoulders

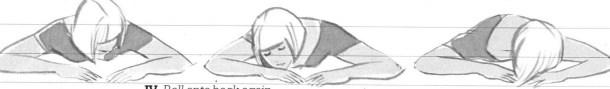

After III, go back to II. Is movement any easier? Once forced feeling goes and muscles relax, movement becomes more fluid...

IV. Roll onto back again. Turn head to one side and keep it there. Lift opposite shoulder towards ceiling several times, then press it firmly into floor several times. Turn head and repeat on other side. Now go back to **I.** Is there any difference?

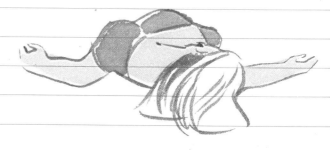

NECK AND SHOULDERS

I. *Place one hand behind the neck so that fingers can feel the muscles along the opposite side. Press index and middle fingers into muscle, rocking head to that side and back to centre as you press and release up and down muscle. Rest a moment.*

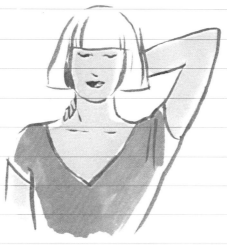

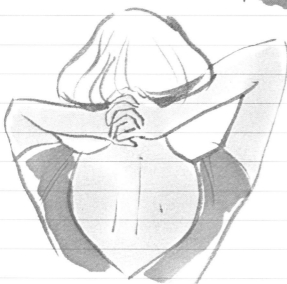

II. *Clasp hands together, interlacing fingers, and massage back, sides and base of neck with heels of hands, pressing firmly and releasing in a gentle rhythm.*

Tension often registers around the base of the neck and shoulders because our natural reaction to stress is to pull in the head and neck. When these muscles tighten up, blood flow to and from the brain may be constricted leading to mental fatigue, headaches and even migraine. Analgesics taken to relieve headache, such as paracetamol (aminocetophen), are often muscle relaxants. They work by reducing tension and so take the pain away. But you can do this for yourself with just massage and gentle exercise.

Help to prevent headaches in the first place with loosening exercises for neck and shoulders and more attention to posture. Your head weighs more than 4.5 kg (10 lb) and should feel *lightly* suspended on your neck, not just dumped on top crushing everything beneath.

III. *Place an orange at back of neck and, gently pressing it between yourself and a wall, roll it around neck, down across shoulders and between shoulder blades, bending and straightening knees, and swaying from side to side. Can you move the orange all the way down to the base of your spine? Enjoy it.*

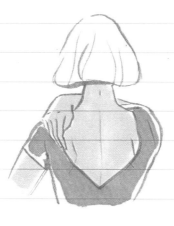

IV. *Place one hand on shoulder and work fingers down towards shoulder blade, pressing them in as far as is comfortable and releasing; then work across shoulder towards arm and back and forth several times. Repeat to other side.*

TO BE FREE OF TENSION BE AWARE OF . . .

Shoulders. Where are they? Hanging freely away from your head or clenched up about your ears?

Breathing. One of the first responses to stress is to hold your breath. This reinforces muscular tension and increases anxiety. Remind yourself to breathe OUT.

Basic body needs. When cramped in the same position for too long muscles are bound to protest. Get up and walk around, shake out arms and legs, stretch in any direction that feels good, breathing out to stretch a little more. Then hang over from the hips letting arms and head drop down, releasing back and allowing blood to run to the brain.

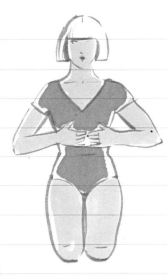

CHEST

Place second, third and fourth fingers of both hands between lower ribs at the front. Breathe in through nose and, as you breathe out, stroke fingers firmly downwards. Repeat several times in a good rhythm, exploring the spaces between your ribs.

Stiffness and tightness in the chest are often indicative of repressed emotion – anger especially and sometimes sadness and grief too. Breathing can help free this area by opening the chest. The pelvic clock exercise (exercise 42 of the main programme) is particularly effective because it encourages you to alternate deep abdominal breathing (6 o'clock) with shallower thoracic breathing (12 o'clock).

SPINE

I. *Lie on floor with knees bent and feet flat. Lift pelvis towards ceiling and then slowly return to floor, unfolding spine vertebra by vertebra. Be aware of your breathing and the quality of the movement. Are you keeping weight evenly on both feet? Repeat several times.*

II. *Lying on floor, with knees bent as before and arms by sides, rock pelvis back and forth between 6 and 12 hands of the pelvic clock, (see page 27). Notice how movement affects position of head and neck.*

III. *Lying as before, raise pelvis towards ceiling again – but not too far. This time visualize two long muscle groups running about 2.5 cm/1 in away from either side of the spine, from the neck to the*

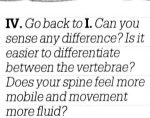

coccyx. Now slowly unroll right-hand side muscles onto floor, making sure waist touches floor before bottom. Notice how pelvis is tilted slightly to that side. Practise several times on same side, then repeat to other side. Which is more agile?

Identify which side of back is more agile.

IV. *Go back to I. Can you sense any difference? Is it easier to differentiate between the vertebrae? Does your spine feel more mobile and movement more fluid?*

SPINE

Lie down on floor and place a soft inflated ball the size of a large grapefruit underneath base of head. Now roll your spine over the ball, pushing with feet, so that you feel you are travelling along the top of it. Take ball up and down in this way a few times. Stop and rest. This affects the very deep muscles of the ribcage and spine. So be gentle. Don't overdo it.

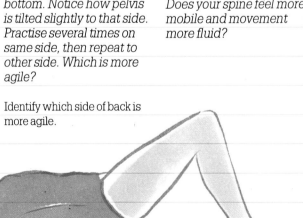

HIPS

I. *Sit as shown. Extend one arm at shoulder level and reach out to side, letting hips move naturally as you go. Return to centre, noticing how hips become level again, and repeat to other side. Repeat several times to each side, rocking gently as you go through centre each time.*

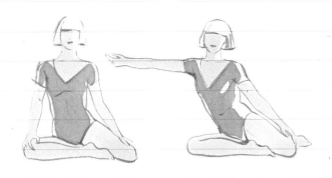

II. *Extend arm to side as before. Now take it round in front of you and over to other side, focusing eyes on hand as it moves so head follows arm naturally round. Then reverse movement and see how far you can go, but don't force it. Repeat several times, then change arms and repeat the exercise.*

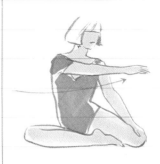

III. *Place one hand on floor beside you. Raise other arm above head and drop head gently back. Return to upright and then lower head and arm as shown. Repeat several times in a good rhythm, noticing what happens to hips and pelvis.*

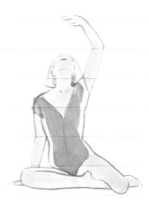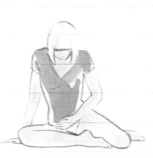

IV. *Place one hand on top of head and tilt it to either side. Notice what happens to hips and pelvis. Repeat a few times, then go back to* **I.** *and* **II.** *Do the movements seem easier? Do you notice an improvement?*

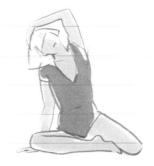

Dancing to Latin or African music is one of the best ways to free the pelvis and loosen the hips because it encourages you to use your body in a sinuous unselfconscious way. Sense movements becoming freer and more fluid as you let yourself go, allowing hips and pelvis to sway and rock and undulate to the rhythms of the music. The best way of freeing the pelvis? Sex!

KNEES

I. *Standing with feet slightly apart, pull up at front of leg so knee feels as though it is being pushed in. Contract firmly several times and repeat several times a day. Many people, women especially, suffer from hyperextension (when knees are pulled back behind the plumbline from hip to arch of foot). This exercise can help to prevent this.*

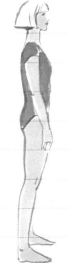

II. *When knee feels stronger, progress to exercise 74 of the main programme, starting without a weight and with thighs well supported on table. Once you can comfortably extend leg, straightening the knee, tie a sock or stocking filled with sand loosely around ankle. Lift slowly and rhythmically up and down several times a day.*

NEVER exercise on a damaged knee; it is a sure way to compound the injury.

When exercising, twisting and rotating movements should come from ankles or hips, not the knee. But if ankles or hips are not sufficiently mobile, the knee may be forced to compensate. Sensations of pain or pulling there, or an apparent lack of flexibility, often reflect stiffness at the joints above and below. Protect your knees by *being aware*. Make sure that they always bend directly over the toes when you exercise, so they are kept in the correct plane and any strain is avoided. If you feel any tension, pressure or twinges of pain, stop working and correct your position. If you find it impossible to do the exercise without straining the knee, leave it for the time being and work instead at increasing mobility at the hips (<u>helpful exercises</u> 42, 111 and 118) and ankles (<u>helpful exercises</u> 17 and 113).
If pain persists, consult your doctor.

PART 2
FAINTNESS

Faintness, light-headedness and sometimes even nausea can accompany exercise – especially if it is vigorous. These sensations are all caused by blood being diverted away from brain and stomach to fuel large muscle groups.

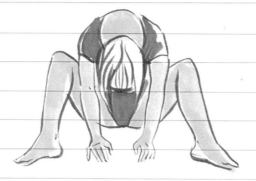

To remedy: stop what you are doing and let blood flow towards brain by placing head lower than rest of body. Either lie on floor or ground with feet up and supported or sit in a chair or on floor, as shown, with legs wide apart and head and arms hanging down between them.

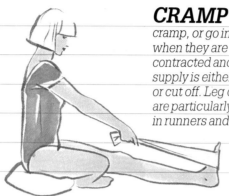

CRAMP
Muscles cramp, or go into spasm, when they are over-contracted and the blood supply is either reduced or cut off. Leg cramps are particularly common in runners and dancers.

STITCH
Stitch, a very sharp pain just below the ribs, is often brought on by unaccustomed exertion – especially running and jumping up and down. Although the exact reason for stitch is not known, it is thought to be caused by lack of oxygen in the respiratory muscles, such as the diaphragm, due to insufficient blood flow. Stitch is soon relieved by stopping and resting and then recommencing activity very gradually. Some distance runners maintain that very deep breathing can sometimes relieve the discomfort while enabling them to continue to run. Try it and see...

I. *As cramped muscles are always over-contracted, stretch muscle out first. When in spasm, resistance is inevitable, so try to enlist the help of someone to hold the leg or arm for you, or use a towel as shown.*

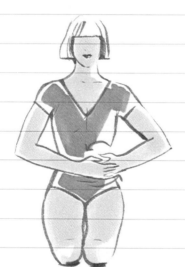

PART 3
HEADACHES

Run through the neck and shoulder loosener sequence first (page 10) and then, if no relief is felt, massage the head itself. Start with forehead.

I. *Close eyes, breathe deeply and check for signs of tension. Release jaw, open brow, let eyes become soft. Place both hands at centre of forehead, just above eyebrows, and stroke firmly outwards. Move up in 3 stages to hairline, and repeat several times.*

II. *Keeping eyes closed, take a few more deep breaths and check again for signs of tension. Now place middle fingers at upper corner of eye just beneath brow, press firmly inwards for count of 5, then release. Repeat this all the way along brow bone to outer corner and then continue underneath the eye. Finish by pressing temples.*

III. *Massage scalp with both hands, working firmly from crown of head backwards.*

STOMACH ACHES
Most digestive problems are caused by stress, manner of eating and diet, in that order. Consider these, especially if you often have digestive problems. Use deep breathing and massage to help increase blood supply to the stomach and ease pain.

I. *Breathe in through nose, filling lungs with air, letting abdomen expand. Hold for a count of 3, then breathe out through mouth drawing abdomen in. This should be slightly longer than the in-breath. Continue in a good rhythm several times.*

II. *Place one hand on top of the other and massage stomach and abdominal area in a clockwise movement.*

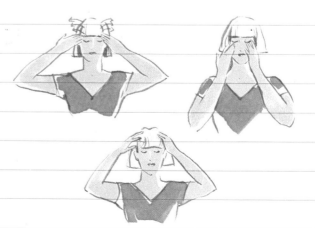

CONSTIPATION

The inverted yoga postures, neck balance (sarvangasana) and plough pose (halasana), can be extremely helpful for digestive problems – relieving abdominal pain and wind and solving constipation especially. In addition, being upside down tends to promote a powerful sense of well-being, clearing the mind and refreshing the system. Practise 5 minutes daily for maximum benefits, but practise with caution: these poses are best learned with the assistance of a professional yoga teacher.

NB If neck or throat feel strained, place folded blanket(s) beneath shoulders, and adjust height and position until comfortable.

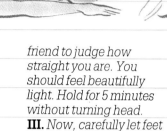
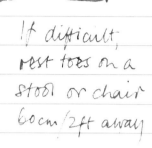

Not when menstruating, or on a full stomach, or if you are high blood pressure

I. *Lie flat on floor, with arms by sides. Take a few deep breaths and bend knees in towards chest till you feel thighs pressing against stomach.*

II. *Raise body up to vertical: move hands down till they are in middle of back and raise hips (only back of head, neck, shoulders and backs of arms up to elbows should now be on floor), stretch legs up and straighten spine. To begin with ask a*

friend to judge how straight you are. You should feel beautifully light. Hold for 5 minutes without turning head.

III. *Now, carefully let feet come over head onto floor to plough pose. Let toes rest on floor, keep legs straight and muscles at front of thighs well pulled up. Extend arms as shown.*

If difficult, rest toes on a stool or chair 60cm/2ft away

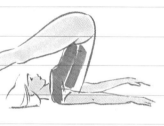

IV. *Cradle knees around head and relax for a moment, before coming out of pose.*

To come out: raise legs to ceiling and slowly lower hips, with help of hands, to ground. Keep movement slow and controlled.

Period Pains

Period pains are caused by strong contractions of the uterine muscles. Tensing up to protect yourself from these contractions makes the pain more intense. Breathing, stretching and curling exercises can help ease pain by encouraging you to relax.

I. *Lie down and breathe deeply several times, trying to focus only on the breath as it enters and leaves your body.*

II. *Raise arms above head, tilt hips to one side and reach up with arms, feeling stretch along side and abdomen. Repeat to other side.*

III. *Curl up knees into abdomen and stay there, breathing well for a few moments. Then stretch out again. Repeat stretch/curl sequence several times.*

IV. *Breathe deeply a few more times, releasing areas of tension and feeling heavier and heavier as you become more and more relaxed.*

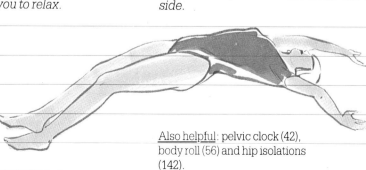
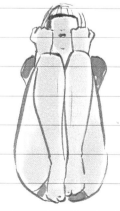

<u>Also helpful</u>: pelvic clock (42), body roll (56) and hip isolations (142).

Index

ACKNOWLEDGEMENTS

The following pictures were taken specially for Octopus Books:
Sandra Lousada 4-5, 107; Butch Martin 99, 100-1, 104; Tom
Wool 1, 2-3, 6-7, 77, 88, 92.

Other photographs are supplied courtesy of *Vogue:* (Jonathan
Lennard) 39, 60; (Butch Martin) 35, 103, 119; (Tom Wool) 17, 25, 69.